Will I DANCE Again?

The Smart Dancers Guide to a Full Recovery from Injury

All rights reserved. No part of this book may be reproduced or transmitted by any person or entity, in any form or by any means, electronic or mechanical, including photocopying, recording, scanning or by any information storage and retrieval system, without prior permission in writing from the publisher.

First published 2014 by

Perfect Form Physiotherapy and The Ballet Blog

Suite 904/121 Walker St, North Sydney, NSW 2060

Copyright © Perfect Form Physiotherapy Pty Ltd 2014

www.perfectformphysio.com.au

www.theballetblog.com

Lisa Howell (B.Phty)

Will I Ever DANCE Again?

Disclaimer:

The contents of this program, including text, graphics, images, videos and other material are for informational purposes only. Nothing contained in this report is or should be considered or used as a substitute for professional medical or health advice, diagnosis, or treatment. The information provided in this report is provided on an "as is" basis, without any warranty, express or implied.

Never disregard medical advice from your doctor or other qualified health care provider or delay seeking it because of something you have read in this document. We urge you to seek the advice of your physician or other qualified health professional with any questions you may have regarding a medical or health condition. In case of emergency, please call your doctor immediately.

Perfect Form Physiotherapy and The Ballet Blog holds no liability or responsibility for any injury or complication that may arise from following this information. Any access to this report is voluntary and at your own risk. If you require further information about any injury please feel free to contact Perfect Form Physiotherapy to organise an individual consultation either in person or via Skype/Phone.

Will I Ever DANCE Again?

Contents

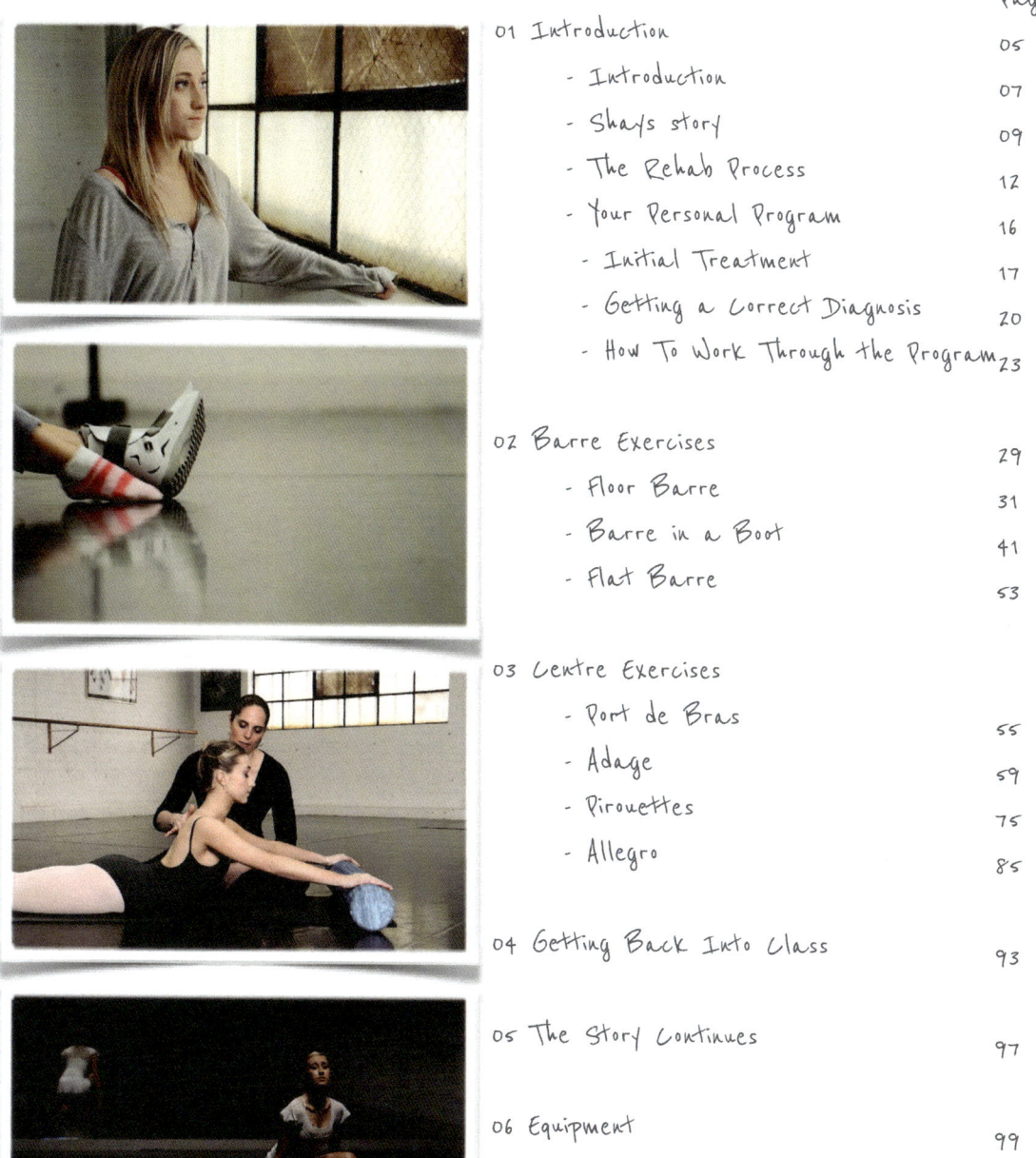

	Page
01 Introduction	05
- Introduction	07
- Shay's story	09
- The Rehab Process	12
- Your Personal Program	16
- Initial Treatment	17
- Getting a Correct Diagnosis	20
- How To Work Through the Program	23
02 Barre Exercises	29
- Floor Barre	31
- Barre in a Boot	41
- Flat Barre	53
03 Centre Exercises	
- Port de Bras	55
- Adage	59
- Pirouettes	75
- Allegro	85
04 Getting Back Into Class	93
05 The Story Continues	97
06 Equipment	99
07 Other Resources	101

Will I Ever DANCE Again?

Introduction

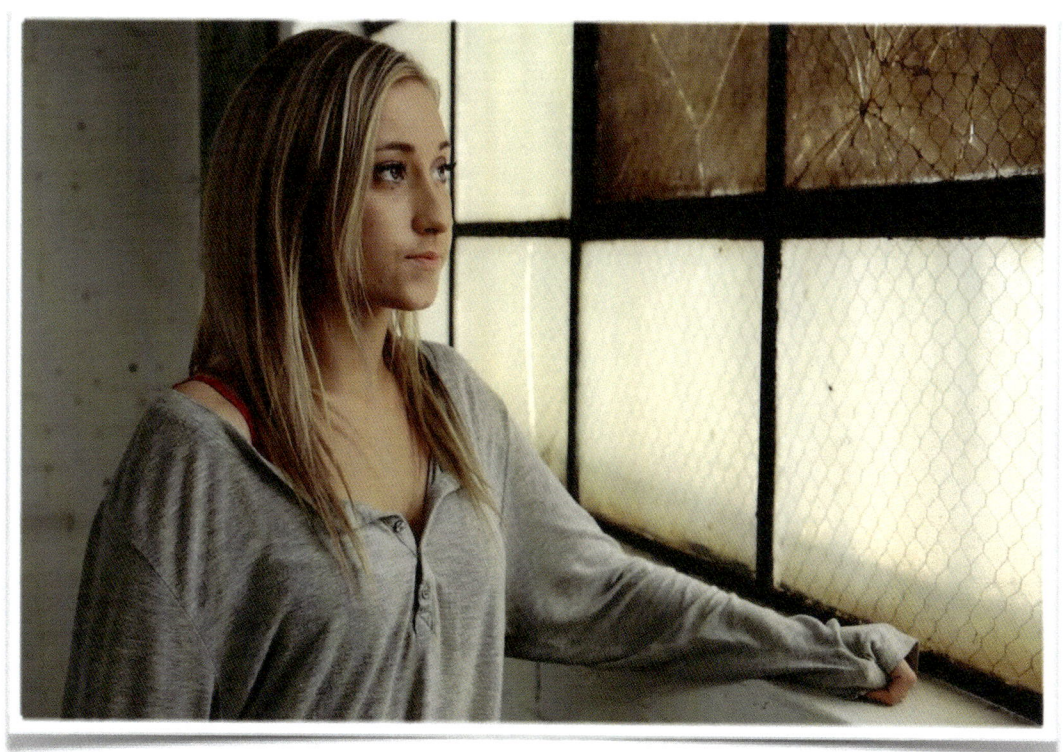

Will I Ever DANCE Again?

Will I Ever DANCE Again?

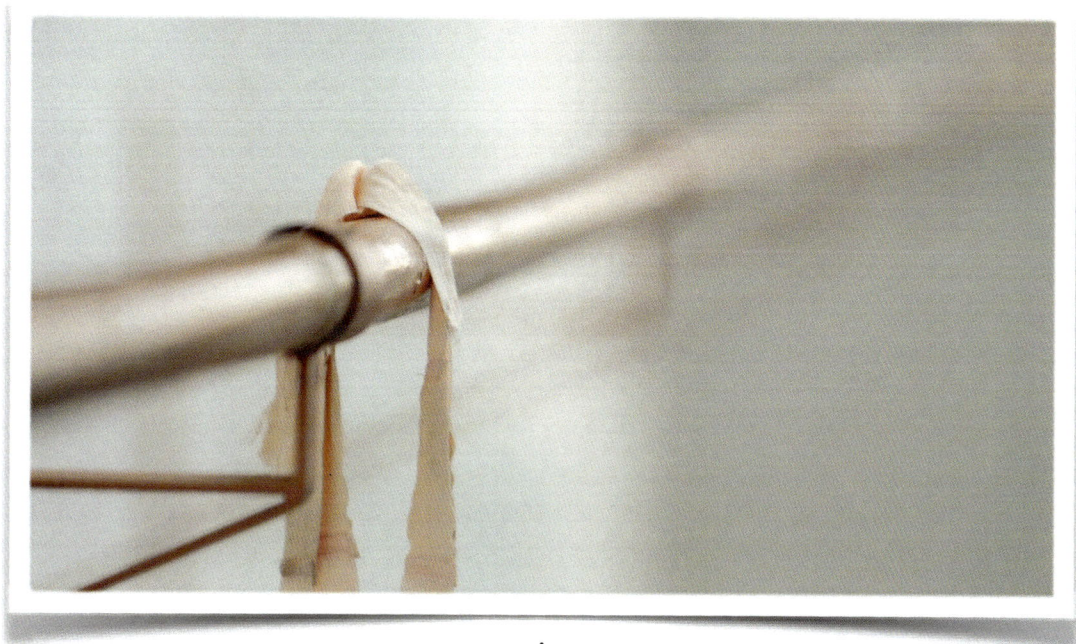

Introduction

If you are a dancer and have been diagnosed with an injury that has forced you to stop dancing, it may feel like your worst nightmare has begun. However, this can actually turn into one of the best experiences, and contribute to your success as a dancer, rather than taking away from it.

After seeing the devastation of chronic injury in so many dancers attempting to dance through injuries that needed time off, and also the success of my clients who had a proper rehab program, I knew I needed to create a guide so that other dancers could do this too, wherever they are in the world. I treat dancers every day, and have produced many resources to help dancers improve their technique as well as prevent and recover from injury. However this program is a little different.

This program starts with a story. A story that simply had to be told. Not because it is unique, but unfortunately, because it is far too common. It is the story of a dancer who thought that her career was over, but who came back stronger, better and more determined, due to a comprehensive and focused rehab program. I hope that this program will help to dispel the voodoo around the meaning of a serious injury to a dancer, and allow more dancers to get back on stage, living their dream.

Will I Ever DANCE Again?

This is the story of one of my students who arrived back in Australia after a career ending injury, at a prestigious pre-professional dance school. It tells of her struggle and her triumphant return to dance, as well as the practical rehab process that we used, and that any dancer can use, to get back into class, and back dancing, stronger and better than ever.

This dancer had a very dramatic and serious injury that forced her to stop dancing. So many dancers actually avoid seeing anyone about an injury that they know is developing because they are scared of taking time off. However this program works on the principle of relative rest in that you can rest the portion of your body that is injured, allowing the natural healing process to work it's magic. Meanwhile you can still participate in class, work the rest of your body, rehabilitate your injury, correct all of the contributing factors that may have caused it, and then return to class in a sensible way. In many cases dancers return to class stronger than before they were injured.

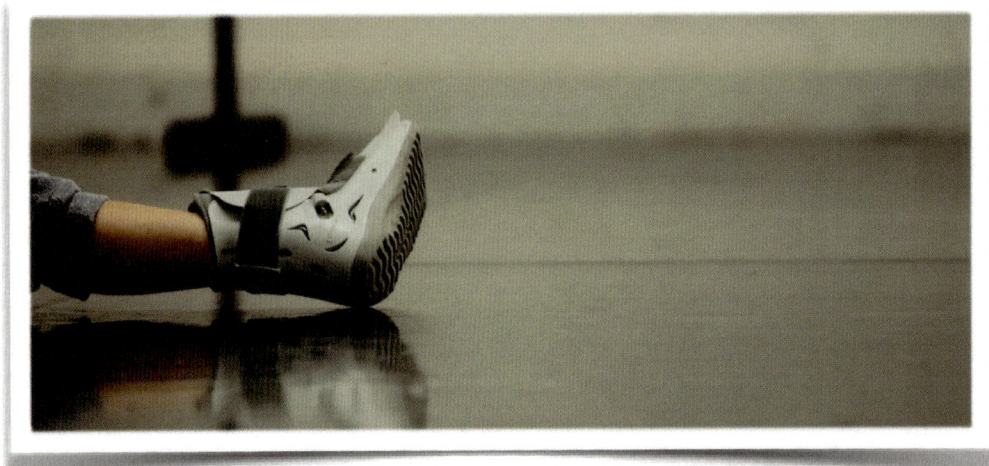

This program is for dancers with acute/traumatic injuries, as well as those dancers who have battled chronic injury, taken time off, and returned to dancing, only to have their pain return. It is also perfect for those with chronic injuries that may have avoided taking time off because of the effect that this will have on their dancing.

My hope is that this program will inspire dancers to undertake the full rehab process, and not be scared to accept an injury, as it can be one of the most powerful gifts a dancer gets. It is a time when you can discover so many ways of improving, learning and growing as an artist, as well as an athlete.

Thank you for sharing our journey.

Will I Ever DANCE Again?

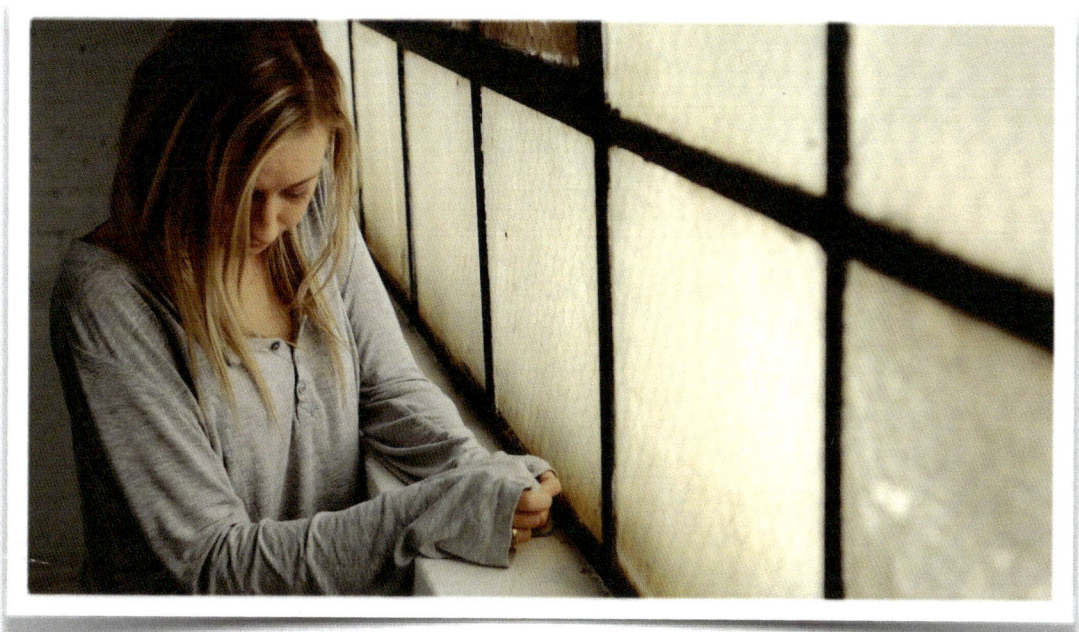

Shay's Story

"Hi, my name is Shayarne Mattheson and I'm a Classical Ballet Dancer. I'm 19 years old and grew up in Sydney, Australia. When I was 3 my mum put me into dance classes. It started off with one a week and then it quickly grew into every afternoon and then I was doing my solo and troupe performances. I just couldn't get enough.

When I was 13 years old thats when I decided that I really wanted to do classical and contemporary dance and I had my mind and my heart set on pursuing it professionally. At 15 I started full time dance and not long after that I went on a European tour to audition for pre-professional schools. I accepted a place in Germany and I was so excited to start.

Not long after that I developed chronic glandular fever and chronic fatigue and I was unable to go. I was on and off dance for a full year sometimes spending weeks at a time bed ridden. I couldn't wait to get back into training. After 4 months of working really hard to get back into peak condition I went to the Alana Haines Awards in New Zealand where I was offered a scholarship to the graduate year of the Royal Ballet School. I couldn't wait to start, I was so excited. I finally felt like I was on my way to achieving my goals and my dreams.

Will I Ever DANCE Again?

I absolutely loved London, I loved training over there, I loved my flat and I made some really wonderful friends while I was there. After only 6 months of training in my normal monday morning ballet class I was doing a petit allegro exercise and came down on my foot wrong. I heard this horrendous snap and immediately thought that my foot was broken.

After I had an X-ray done we realised it wasn't broken and it was treated as a sprain. After a couple of weeks of absolutely no improvement the decision was made for me to come home. I was absolutely devastated. When I got home we diagnosed my injury. It was far worse than a sprain. I was immediately put on crutches and started my rehab program with Lisa.

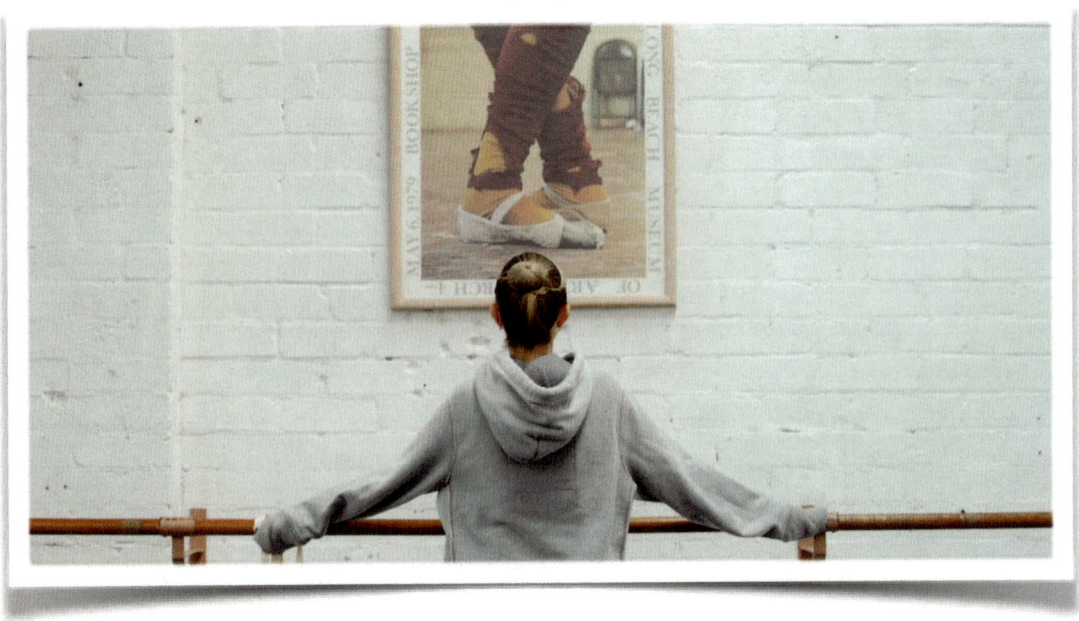

I should have gone into a boot straight away but I fought it and fought it because to me being in a boot meant that it was real and I was seriously injured.

I was finally convinced to get into a boot which just changed everything. My mental state went from being absolutely awful, I was devastated and didn't know whether I was ever going to dance again to things changing completely. I got my independence back, I was able to get myself around and I was even able to get back into class. That including the fact that I could have my foot supported and still go to the gym to keep my cardio up as well as my rehab program just changed everything. I finally felt like I was back on track.

Will I Ever DANCE Again?

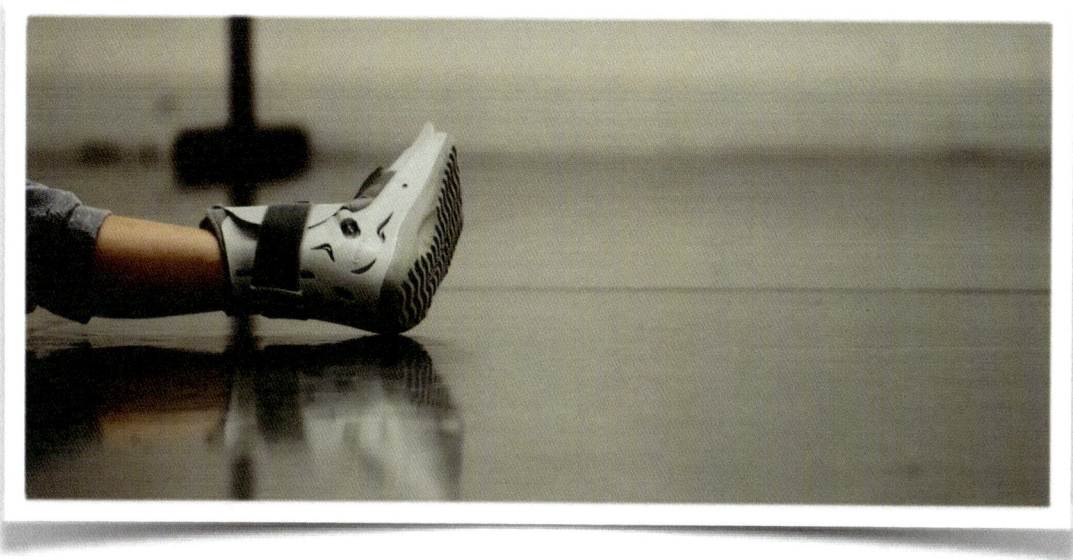

It just proves that if you have the right mind set and you take the right steps that you can bounce back from anything no matter how difficult you thought it would be, and you can come back better for it.

Im really glad that this injury has not only helped myself but now we can use it to help other dancers who have gone through similar situations get back to what they love doing most."

Shayarne Mattheson

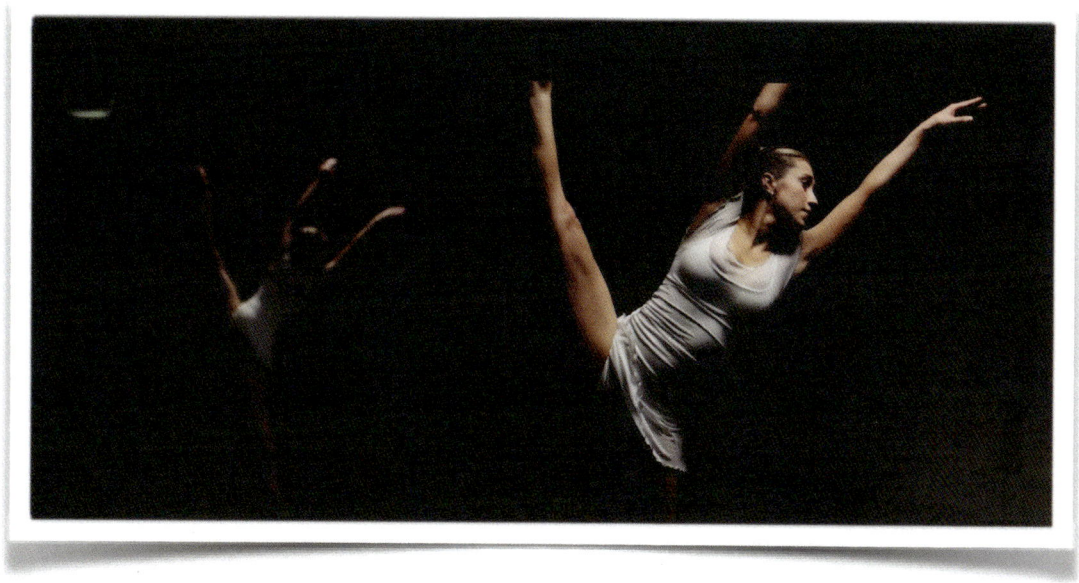

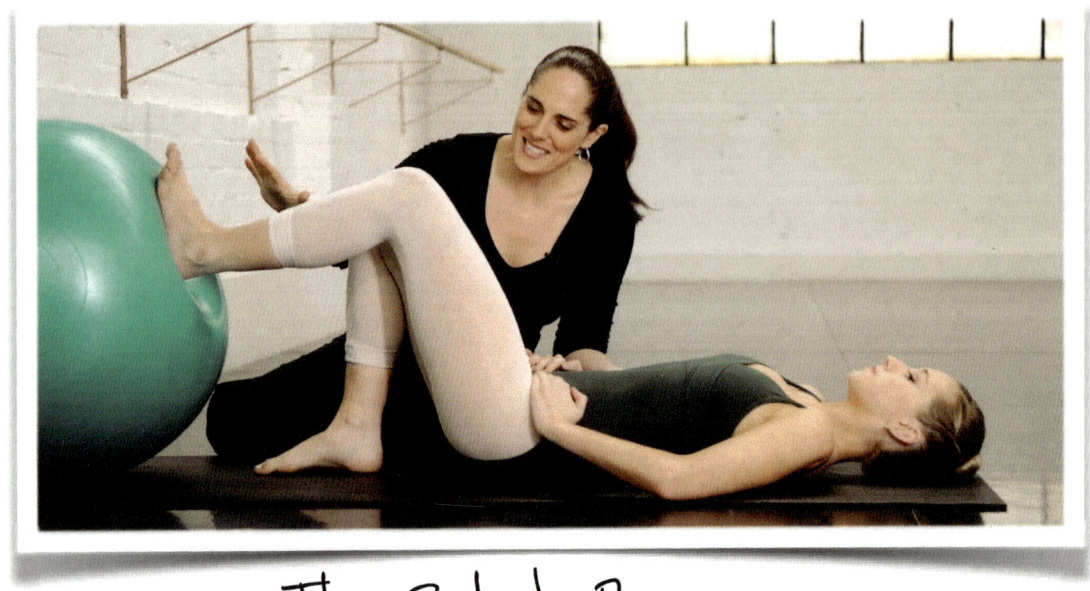

The Rehab Process

This program is all about maintaining and improving your technique while you are injured, and correcting all of the contributing factors, to get you back into class as soon as possible. This is usually not a full class, but you should able to do a modified class depending on what kind of injury you have. This program focuses mainly on foot injuries, as these are the injuries that seem to worry dancers the most, however, you can use modifications of these exercises for almost any other injury that you have. (Details of these are online in the Members Area of The Ballet Blog)

It is obviously very important to treat any injury directly, but part of that treatment should also be avoiding any further injury. The focus is to give the injured area relative rest while still continuing to train the rest of the body. This is to make sure that you maintain and improve strength in all other areas. Having a little time off your full dancing schedule is a great opportunity to improve on areas of your technique that you find difficult, and especially those areas that may have lead to your injury developing in the first place.

One of the most powerful reasons why we need to get you back in class is the psychological impact that stopping dancing can have on a dancer. When what you do is so enmeshed with your perception of who you are, having that removed from your life can challenge the very deepest parts of you.

Will I Ever DANCE Again?

A serious injury, especially a foot injury that requires a significant period of time off dancing, can start a dangerously slippery slope of doubting your ability to get back, perhaps a fear of putting on weight, of losing condition or perhaps even contemplating the possibility of never being able to dance again.

This is one reason why dancers who start to become aware of an injury developing often ignore the early warning signs, because they are so scared of what time off will mean to their career.

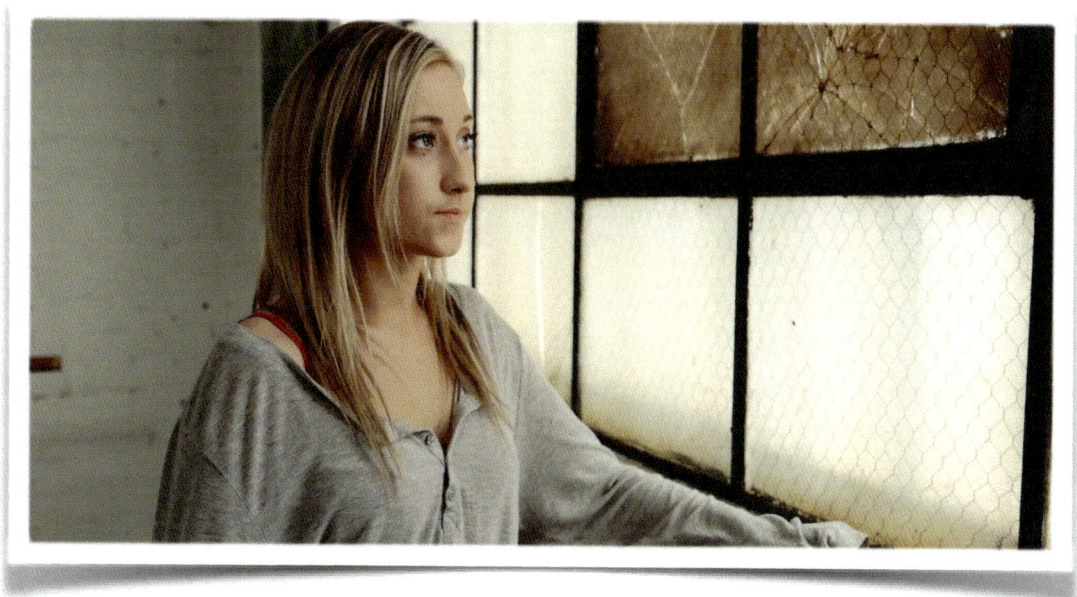

The truth of the matter is that most students I work with on this kind of program actually end up thankful for their injury. They learn so much about their body, and themselves, during the rehab process, that they return to dance not only stronger physically but also with less fear of injury. They feel empowered that they can recover from whatever is thrown at them in the future.

The psychological benefit of getting back into class and working on a structured program that is aimed at healing rather than continuing to harm is massive. However, it may not be right for everyone. I have found some students tend to rehab better alone, outside the studio, because they don't like being in class unless they are at full capacity. However, these students are definitely the minority, so please do try the variations of normal class exercises within the class environment to see how it works for you.

Will I Ever DANCE Again?

Correct Contributing Factors

One of the most important factors in any rehab program is identifying and correcting any contributing factors that led to that injury developing in the first place. This is especially important when dealing with chronic injuries that keep re-occurring.

One of the biggest things that we need to look at with this is your turnout and your core control, as many foot and ankle injuries occur due to rolling in of the supporting foot, or over-bracing with the tendons around the ankle. However, in this program we will not be going over all of the specific exercises for these as we have gone over them a lot in some of our other programs. Please consult the Appendix at the back of this book for suitable exercises that may be included from other programs.

It is important to carry through all of the isolated strengthening to your class work to correct any habits that have formed over the years, such as rolling in or over turning the supporting foot. Any time off dancing should be focused on maximising strength, mobility and control in all other areas, rather than wasting away your hard earned strength.

Overall A General Rehab Process Should:

- Start with a period of relative rest or non weight-bearing, depending on the injury
- Focus on correct isolation of all muscles
- Improve co-ordination and strength around the core and hips
- Include a gradual and graded transition back into class
- Retrain the motor patterns required for optimal movements
- Result in the dancer being stronger than before the injury!

Will I Ever DANCE Again?

The Structure of the Program

The rehab process usually starts off with a period of non weight-bearing, which varies in time depending on the exact injury that you have. You may be in a boot, or you may just need to have the foot taped and be on crutches while the injury heals. It is also very important to maintain your cardiovascular fitness during this time, so please see our suggestions in the online Members Area for ideas.

During this time you really want to focus on specific isolation of the muscles around the core, the hips and in the feet to keep the rest of you moving. If you have to be non weight-bearing then you can use the floor barre routine to help keep all of your other muscles working. You may also need to use a floor barre in the early stages in a boot if the injury is very vulnerable, or if the boot is too heavy for you to lift at the barre.

Please also remember that a floor barre is a very powerful training tool for any dancer, even when you are not injured, and should be used at least once a week in addition to your normal class work.

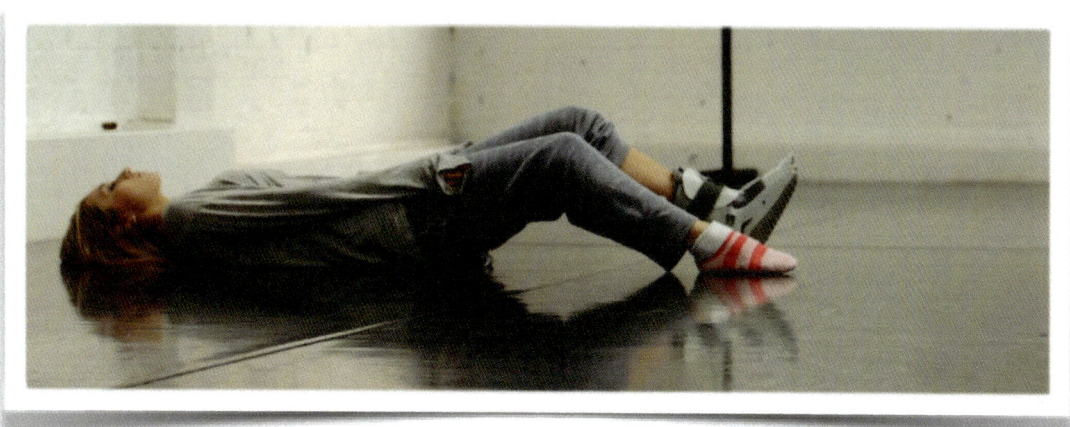

For those of you that are allowed to weight-bear but must have the foot supported, Shay will demonstrate how a dancer can participate in class when wearing a boot. I will also discuss working with a flat barre which is a wonderful training tool to use when you are allowed to build back into class. For your centre work, I have given some non weight-bearing variations. Then I will go through a progressive set of exercises to help you build back into class work once you are allowed to take weight through the foot again.

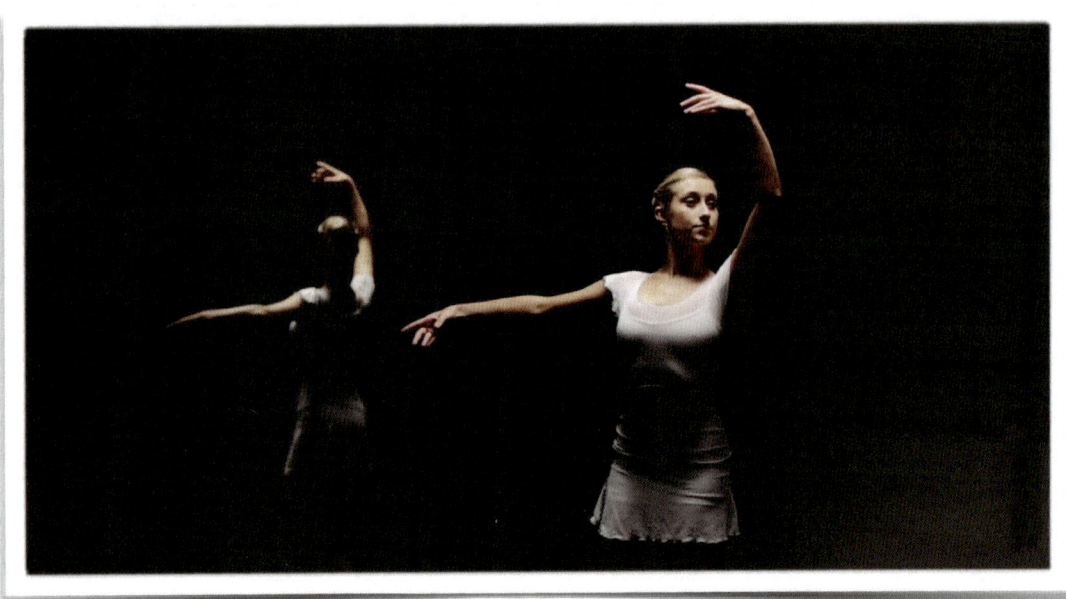

Your Personal Program

There is so much more to the ultimate care of your injury than just the exercises that you do when you are in class. Please take some time to read and watch through all of the information in the online Members Area to make sure that all other aspects of your rehab are correctly laid out. Things that you need to think about include:

- Initial Treatment
- Getting A Correct Diagnosis
- How To Work Through The Program
- What To Do If You Don't Have A Dance Physio
- How To Warm Up Properly
- Cardio Training for Dancers
- Your Daily Program
- Building Back Into Class

All of these things should be discussed with your treating therapist, so make sure that you ask them what is appropriate for you at each stage of your rehabilitation. Remember that this book is just a guide to help you and your therapist make sure that you address all parts of your rehab properly. It is not a substitute for a therapist.

Will I Ever DANCE Again?

Initial Treatment

> Everyone has had one of those moments where you come down on your foot wrong in class or worse yet, you're doing something completely unrelated to dance and you go over on your ankle and immediately know that something is really wrong. However, there are several things that you can do right at the point of injury that can make a big difference to how long it takes for you to get back into class.

1. Breathe

Often when you tumble to the ground and you're in pain or you've got the shock of falling, this will increase your heart rate. As your heart rate increases this can increase swelling and bruising and you want to minimise this as much as possible. You may think that there is nothing you can do to stop the immediate reaction to get upset, but there is! With practice you can learn to centre yourself a whole lot more effectively when something like this happens.

The first thing you should do if you have an injury is to close your eyes. Focus on your heart and your breathing rate and see if you can will both of them to slow down. It's a good idea to practice this at home at other times as this will then come more naturally when you do actually have an injury.

2. Don't be a hero

Usually the first thing that you want to do when you fall over with an injury is to get back up and keep on dancing. It is important not to do this as when you've just had a fall and possibly gone into shock, you'll have higher levels of adrenaline in your system. Adrenaline is a chemical that we have evolved to use in stressful situations that allows us to keep on going. However if you continue to keep dancing on an unstable ankle or knee you're much more likely to re-injure that area or make the injury worse. It's important to stop, calm yourself and make sure that everything is ok before coming back into class if it's safe to do so.

One of the reasons why many people want to jump back into class is that they're worried that their teacher thinks they're being slack by taking time out. However I've talked to a lot of teachers about this and the majority of them would much rather that you take some time out and assess what's going on rather than dancing through an injury.

Will I Ever DANCE Again?

3. Assess the damage

Next, assess what is going on to determine the next step. If it's an ankle injury, gently point and flex the foot, or sickle it in and out to see where it hurts. The important thing is to do this testing yourself, using your own muscles rather than having someone else do it for you. What you are trying to find out what structures are actually damaged and how badly.

If there's a lot of pain you should immobilise it, however if its just a slight pain when you start doing these movements then you may try placing weight through the foot to see if there is an increase of pain with pressure.

4. R.I.C.E

R.I.C.E stands for Rest, Ice, Compression and Elevation. This is important in the initial stages of some injuries to help reduce excessive swelling. However, do remember that swelling is natural process that is designed to flood the injured area with lots of blood cells and fluid to heal the injury. The fluid and swelling also helps to immobilise the joint so that you don't re-injure it. You don't want to stop the swelling completely, but if you have too much stagnant swelling this can interfere with your healing and treatment later on.

Rest - This is obvious, don't continue to walk around or dance on it if it's quite sore. You want to take time out from class.

Ice – It's very important that you apply ice correctly. A lot of people take one ice pack, pop it on and leave it there for a couple of hours and then forget about it. This is not what you need to do! Ideally get a fluid ice pack (e.g some ice cubes in a bag of water) that will mould around the joint rather than using a hard ice pack on one part of the joint. Apply the ice pack between 10-20 min depending on the size of the area and the severity of the injury. Then remove it for 20 mins before putting it back on. Continue to have the ice on and off the area for the next 24-48 hours depending on the severity of the injury. This will allow new blood flow to keep coming into the area whilst preventing too much fluid from staying in the area.

Will I Ever DANCE Again?

Compression – You can apply some compression with a gentle bandage but make sure not to wind it up too tight. Keep an eye on your toes to make sure that they don't turn white or blue!

Elevation – It's not enough to pop your foot up on a bag. Your foot should be above your knee, which is above your hip to allow the fluid to come back down into your lymphatic system and reduce swelling.

5. Get professional advice

I cannot stress this enough! Even if you think you've just got a "normal" ankle injury, it is very important to make sure it is actually a simple ankle sprain and that you have your treatment plan on track. There are a lot of things that can make a seemingly simple injury very complicated and slow to heal and it's much better to find those out in the beginning rather than several weeks later.

For example, with an ankle sprain, there are several common issues that require different treatment, that may look like a lateral sprain. If you have a Syndesmotic injury (an injury to the ligament that helps hold the 2 bones of the lower leg together) this must be dealt with very specifically. Alternatively if you have an an Avulsion Fracture (where the muscle pulls a little chunk of bone off its attachment point) the earlier we know about it the better.

6. Listen to the advice!

The most important thing is to actually listen to the advice form your healthcare professional! Far too often people go to see a therapist but then go against what the therapist asks them to do and end up re-injuring themselves. If the therapist asks you to do something that you don't want to do or don't think is right, ask them more questions about it and clarify why it is that you should be doing that. If you really insist on pushing through with a major performance please tell them that you're going to do it so that they can at least tape you to prevent further damage rather that doing it behind their back!

Please be honest with your therapist as it is only then that they can help you the most!

Will I Ever DANCE Again?

Getting a Correct Diagnosis

One of the most important factors before commencing any rehabilitation program is getting a correct diagnosis. Especially in Shay's Story we learnt how important this is in getting you into the right rehab program from the very beginning. Please consult a qualified medical professional to get a detailed diagnosis and treatment plan, and follow their guidance throughout the whole rehab process. Getting this right from the beginning can save you weeks, or even months of rehabilitation.

A correct diagnosis will let you know exactly what structures are injured, and how badly, so that you know what must be rested, and what can be used. For every injury there are a different set of requirements.

- For Shays injury – a major **ligament injury** in the mid-foot, it was important that we immobilise her foot in a boot, but we could allow a little movement at the ankle

- If there is an issue with the **Achilles tendon**, or perhaps a **posterior impingement** or an **Os Trigonum** removal, then you may be restricted from pointing the foot for a period of time

- If there is an issue with the tendon that goes to the big toe **(Flexor Hallucis Longus),** you may only be able to pointe the foot to a demi point position

- **Stress fractures** of the lower leg or foot may need some time in a boot, or a period of non weight-bearing (on crutches) however this is not always necessary

Please Note: This program is not intended to diagnose or treat any injury. However it can help dance teachers who desperately want to keep their students in shape, yet are fearful of pushing their students too hard. It can help dance teachers work with their injured students safely rather than watching them slump depressed in the corner as their class mates dance.

It can also help health professionals with no dance training understanding the demands of a dance class to create an ordered progressive way of getting their clients back to what they love doing most.

Will I Ever DANCE Again?

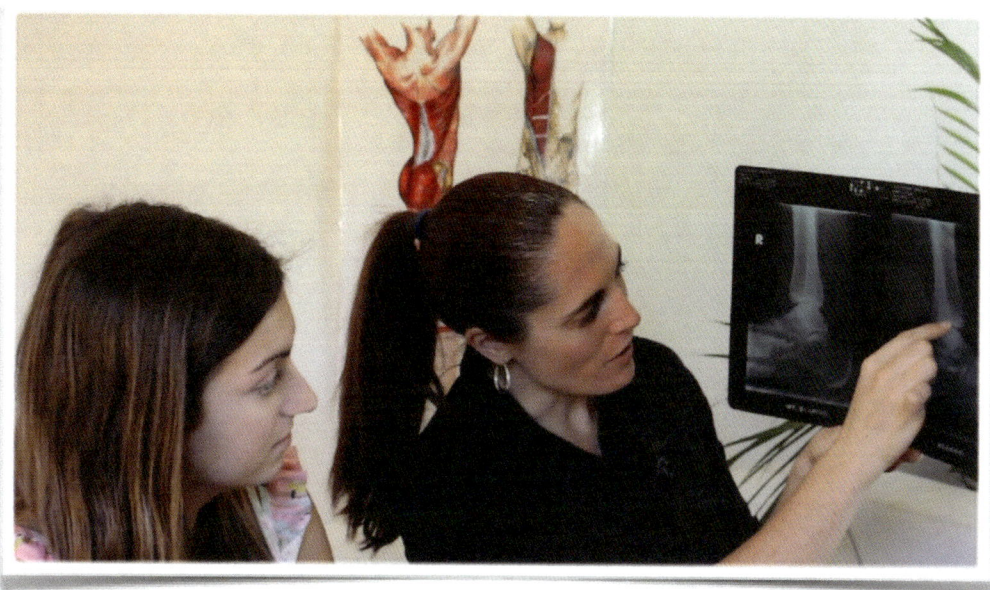

Use the following points and questions to work with your therapist to get a clear plan in place for your rehab.

1. Trust Yourself

- You are the one who is experiencing the injury so when you are given a diagnosis, make sure that their explanation matches what you are feeling

- If it does not, ask more questions until it feels right

2. Make sure that the injury isn't actually something else

- When you first go to see a Therapist or Doctor they will ask you a lot of questions to try to work out what is going on

- They should then do a series of specific tests to determine what structures are injured so that they can work out the most appropriate treatment

- Get them to write down exactly what they think your diagnosis is

- Must be a "differential diagnosis" between all of the different conditions that can give pain in the same area

- Ask them what it is NOT

Will I Ever DANCE Again?

3. Find out what structures are involved and how long to heal

- Does your injury involve the bone, cartilage, tendon, muscle or a combination of several structures? This will really help determine the most effective and efficient treatment and rehab plan
- Ask what the normal healing time-frame would be. Remember that this can be a very hard question to answer!

4. "How can I assist the healing?"

- Therapists love this question!
- Things that you can do may involve dietary changes, icing, contrast bathing or compressive bandages etc
- May need to load the area to make sure that the fibres of the muscle or tendon align properly

5. "What am I allowed to do?"

- Check with your therapist whether you are allowed to walk, swim, do each type of dance class, or climb stairs, as It is very important to continue training the rest of your body. Just because you have injured one foot does not mean that you can't work the other one
- Also get a list of what you must NOT do
- You may need to tape your foot off your full pointe range when swimming to avoid compressing the back of the ankle if you have Posterior Impingement

6. "Do I need to get any X-rays or other scans done?"

- This is often not needed – so do not worry if they say no!
- We want to limit the amount of radiation that you are exposed to
- However, scans can helpful if it is a very difficult, complicated injury, or one that is slow to heal
- You must not rely solely on the scan reports to diagnose an injury

Will I Ever DANCE Again?

How To Work Through The Program

> There is a **HUGE** amount of information in this program, so I wanted to give you a little orientation on how to get the most out of it. There are a **LOT** of exercises in the program, but please do not let this daunt you. You will not be doing them all at once! However I do advocate a pretty intensive rehab program, so you will not be slacking off when doing this program!

1. You **MUST** also make sure that you have been to see a qualified doctor, Sports Physician, Physiotherapist, Physical Therapist or Osteopath to get an accurate diagnosis (what is wrong) and prognosis (how long it should take to heal). **THIS IS ESSENTIAL TO GETTING AN EFFECTIVE REHAB PROGRAM IN PLACE.** This program is ideal for keeping the rest of your body, and your dancing technique, up to scratch, however everyone will need slightly different specific exercises, stretches and treatment for the part that is actually injured.

2. The next thing to do is to read/watch all of the introductory posts and videos, preferably in order. This will give you a deeper understanding of how to actually structure your day and include the program into your life.

3. Watch through the program, but please do not do any exercises until you have cleared them with your therapist. Some injuries require different treatment than others, and it is impossible to outline them all here. Doing an exercise too early could set you back several weeks in your rehab, so this is very important.

4. Show the program with your therapist and discuss your rehab plan with them to determine **what components you are allowed to do each week**. For instance, if you are put in a boot for a fracture, you may be only able to do a floor barre with your non injured foot initially, with the other foot in a boot on a pillow until it is stable enough to walk on.

5. Discuss what **cardiovascular training** options are suitable for you at the moment, and when you will be able to add in other things. For instance, if you have just had surgery, you need to wait until the scars are fully closed before going into a pool, due to the risk of infection if any water enters the surgical scar.

6. **Set up your schedule** around whatever other commitments you have, i.e. school, work etc. Remember that I advocate doing **at least half** the amount of hours that you normally train (uninjured) on your rehab. So, if you normally train over 30 hours a week, you must do at least 15 hours or dedicated rehab every week. This can be increased up to your normal hours as long as you have good technique, and a well rounded program. The specific strengthening can be quite intense, and you do not want to get any overuse injuries by doing too much rehab too quickly!

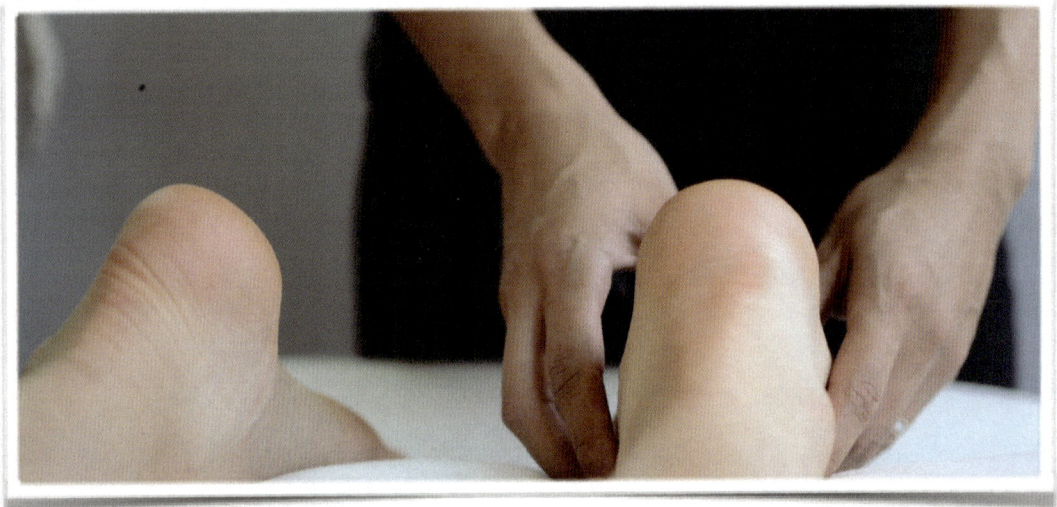

7. **Follow your Surgeon, Doctor or Therapists advice over anything in this DVD.** They will know the exact details of your injury and can guide you through the process. This program is designed to give you options, and help maintain the rest of your body while the injured portion heals, but taking care of the injury has the highest priority.

8. Usually, if you have an acute foot or ankle injury, or have just had surgery, you will need to stick to all of the **"Non Weight-Bearing"** options for each section of class first. Please take note of the variation that you must do, i.e. foot fully flexed, loosely pointed, pointing to demi pointe only or fully pointed. A sample program may include the following exercises:

- Floor Barre – Plie, Battement Tendu, Battement Fondu etc
- Port de Bras – on a chair, foot elevated
- Adage – Cushion Squeezes, Thoracic Sliding, Parallel to Turnout
- Allegro – Gluteal Firing
- Pirouettes – Knee Openings, Standing Leg Turnout

9. If you are in a boot, but not allowed to put weight through it yet, or the boot is too heavy for you to use in standing, please keep the boot on, with the foot and leg resting on a pillow, and do the floor barre with the other leg only. You may need to place the leg with the boot through a doorway to allow the other foot to be placed on the wall.

10. If you are in a boot and allowed to put weight through it, you **MUST** check with your therapist before starting any of the exercises. However, you may be able to do a program including:

- Barre with a Boot
- Port De Bra – on a ball, boot on
- Adage – Cushion Squeezes, Thoracic Sliding, Stingray
- Allegro – Gluteal Firing, Heel Press
- Pirouettes – Knee Openings

11. If you are allowed to walk on your foot, but not allowed to rise, you may be able to add in exercises such as a Flat Barre, Proprioception Exercises or Balance In Retire

12. Once you are allowed to rise, but not jump, then adding in progressions such as Preparation for Petit Jeté, and some single leg rises may be added

13. To build endurance and control before returning fully to class, make sure that you can master the higher level exercises such as the Preparation for Grande Jeté, and Preparation for Pirouette to challenge all of your stability muscles.

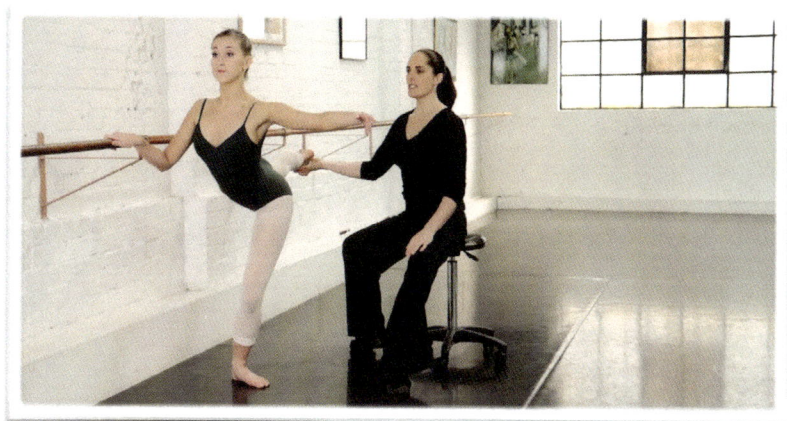

Will I Ever DANCE Again?

What To Do If You Don't Have A Dance Physio

> While it does help if your therapist knows a little (or a lot) about exactly what is involved in a ballet class, and also the psychological pressures that often come with a dance injury, just because your therapist is not a dancer, or used to treating dancers, does not mean that you are in bad hands! There are some absolutely amazing therapists in the world who have never done a dance class in their life, and can still treat you very, very well, so just because they do not advertise that they work with dancers, please do not write them off!

Obviously, if you do have access to a great physio who is used to working with dancers then this is wonderful, as they will be able to help you to recover from your current injury, but can also help you refine your technique to help prevent the injury from re-occurring (especially if it was a chronic injury) . With a carefully tailored program they can also help improve your strength, mobility and technique in other areas, to make sure that you return to dance actually better than you were before the injury. If you are in an area where you do not have access to a good dance physio, you can contact us at the clinic for a Skype consultation, or use the following tips to help your current therapist treat you as efficiently as possible.

1. Show them what you need to be able to do – most good therapists have an ability to analyse movement, and see what is needed to rebuild the strength needed to perform it, no matter what the activity. Take in photos of you dancing, and videos if possible, from before you were injured so that they can see what level you are at, and exactly what you need to get back to.

2. Help them redefine 'normal' – The 'normal' ranges of motion that apply to regular people simply do not apply to most dancers. You train your body constantly to push the boundaries of what is humanly possible, so do not be surprised if the therapist thinks its amazing that you can touch your toes! Make sure that they understand what is 'normal' for you, by comparing to your other side, or how you were before the injury. For instance, they might be very happy with getting a torn hamstring back to 120 degrees, when you know that you need to get it to 160 for a certain performance piece.

Will I Ever DANCE Again?

3. Use our injury reports – We are slowly compiling a series of injury reports that outline the causes, contributing factors, treatment protocol and rehab process for many common dance injuries. Please check out the selection of these injury reports in The Ballet Blog online store. Print out the appropriate report and take it along to your therapist so that they can get an idea of what is expected in a rehab program for this kind of injury. If you have purchased the **Advanced Foot Control for Dancers** program, all of these reports will be in the Members Area, and for anyone else, or for hip, knee and back injuries, they can be purchased individually.

4. Use a floor barre - Hopefully your teacher will have some experience in using a simple floor barre to help you stay in condition if you do have to be off your feet for a period of time. If they don't, then please show them the one that we use here. This is especially needed after foot or ankle surgery, stress fractures and recent ligament injury. It is however essential that you modify the floor barre for whatever injury you have. For example, if you have had an Os Trigonum removed from the back of your ankle, you will not be able to pointe the foot in tendus. If you have had a hip injury, you may not be able to do floor barre lying on your back, as this can overload the front of the hips.

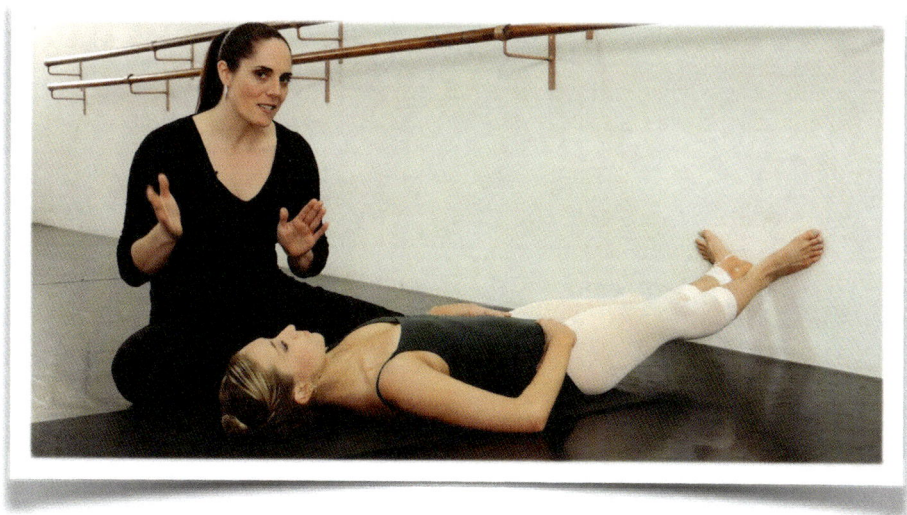

5. Correct all of the contributing factors – these reports should help your therapist assess you in enough detail to work out many of the contributing factors to the injury developing in the first place. This is a hugely important part in developing and effective rehabilitation program. You must correct each of the contributing factors (such as rolling in due to a lack of turnout control) to help prevent re-injury when you return to class

6. Break down each exercise – If you are unable to stand, it is important to train all of the components of each exercise that you do in standing, in order to not lose condition in that area, whether or not that is related to your actual injury. For instance, if you are unable to balance on one foot due to a stress fracture on that side, it is very important that you continue to train all of the muscles that you would normally use in adage to maintain and even improve them.

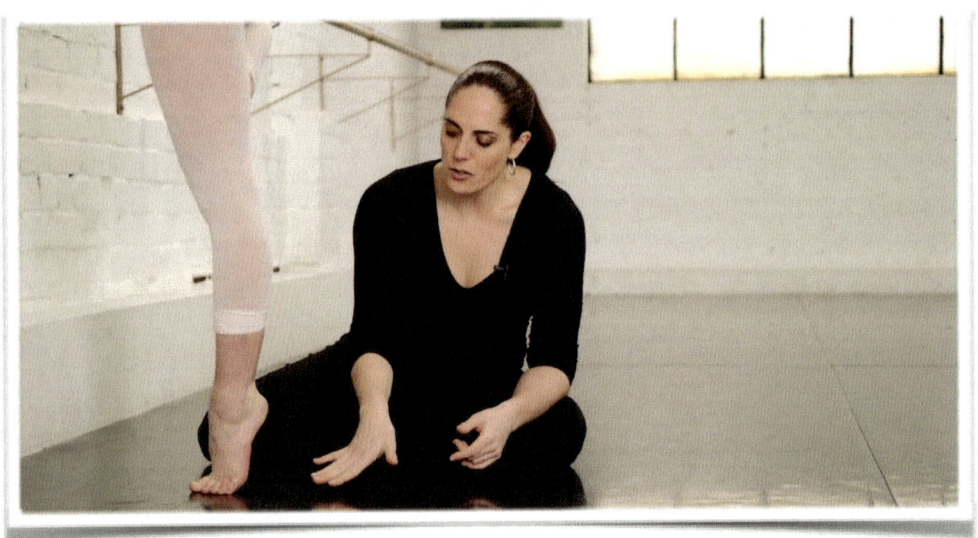

This is where it does get a little tricky for some therapists, and it is also hard for dance teachers, who may know the steps, but not the specifics of exactly what muscles need to be trained to really improve a particular step, or the modifications of some exercises for each different injury.

This is why we have created this program, that outlines the complete rehab process of a dancer, from complete non weight-bearing, to working in class in a boot and then finally building back into full class in a safe and sensible way. "Will I Ever Dance Again?" helps improve your confidence, by dropping the fear of re-injury as progress is gradual and tailored to your specific injury. You will also actually improve your technique in many areas, as each section of class is broken down and includes carefully chosen exercises to improve the strength, flexibility, coordination and balance needed to execute each step properly.

The program can be used by any dancer, under the guidance of their treating therapist, who has had at least 5 years of formal dance training. It is modelled around the structure of a normal classical class so that you can still participate in class during your rehab process.

Barre Exercises

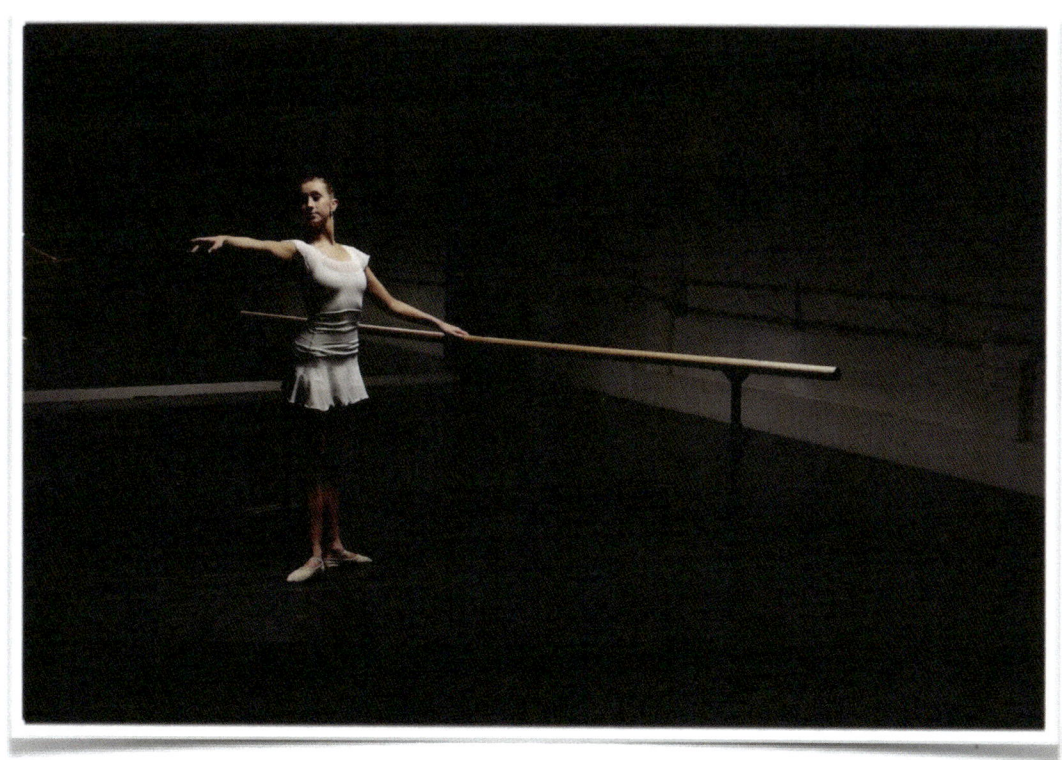

Will I Ever DANCE Again?

Will I Ever DANCE Again?

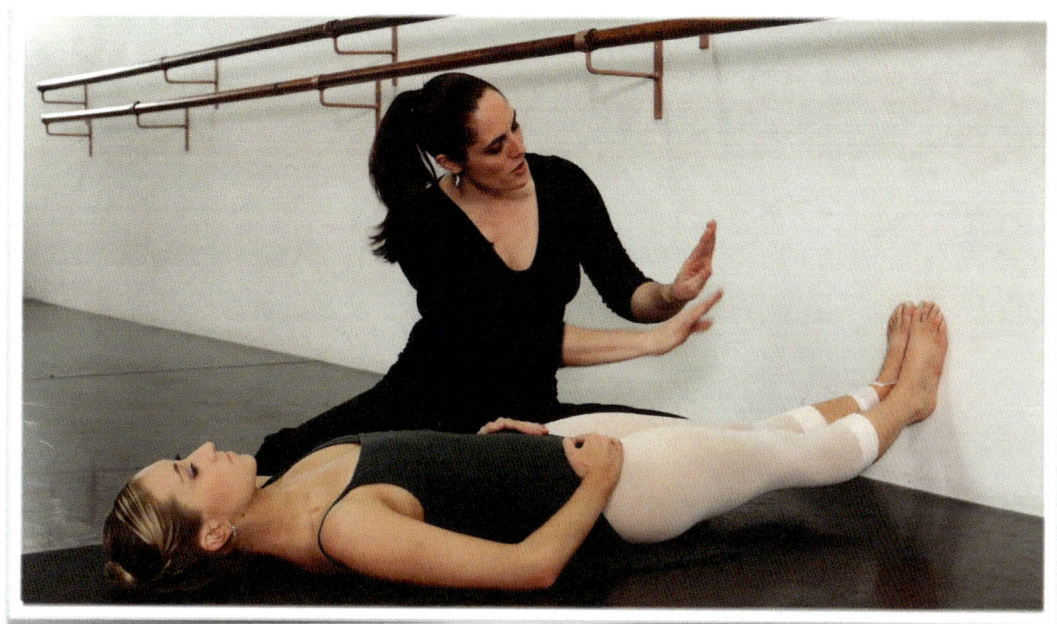

Floor Barre

A floor barre is a fantastic way of maintaining core, hip, and foot control whilst not weight-bearing on your feet, for instance when recovering from a stress fracture or surgery. It is often more challenging than a normal barre and is an effective way of improving your technique whilst you are not allowed to do normal classwork. While doing floor barre you can often quickly work out where your weaknesses lie and you may also discover discrepancies in strength or range of motion from side to side.

Floor barre can be done in the comfort of your own home, at the gym or in your normal ballet class, where you can follow the structure of the class with your classmates.

Just like any dance class, it is important to warm up effectively before starting a floor barre. Make sure your warm up includes some spinal mobility exercises, hip mobilisers and a foot warm up. It is also important to include some isolation and activation exercises for your core, turnout, deep inner thigh and intrinsic foot muscles. For more information and a sample warm up please visit the online Members Area on The Ballet Blog.

For all floor barre exercises you can choose to do either 4-8 repetitions of the demonstrated exercise, or follow along with your syllabus work. However, if performing these exercises to music please make sure to slow down to half speed if there is a particularly fast exercise.

Will I Ever DANCE Again?

Floor Barre - Set Up

Once you have warmed your body up and performed some basic activation exercises of your feet, adductors, core and turnout, it is time to begin setting yourself up for floor barre. It is important to take time to set up properly to ensure that you are using the correct muscles. Take your time with this exercise and take note if you feel or can see any differences on one side compared to the other.

1. Start by lying flat on your back and place your feet in parallel approximately 10cm up the wall. This should allow for the alignment of your legs to replicate a normal standing posture. It is important not to have your heels on the floor.

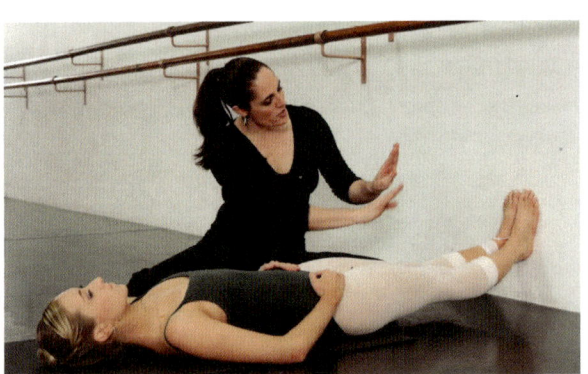

2. Your spine should be in neutral, meaning you maintain a small curve in your lower back. This curve should be just enough to allow the front of your pelvis to be horizontal. Lengthen through the back of your neck and widen through the front of your chest. Gently activate your core muscles to maintain this position.

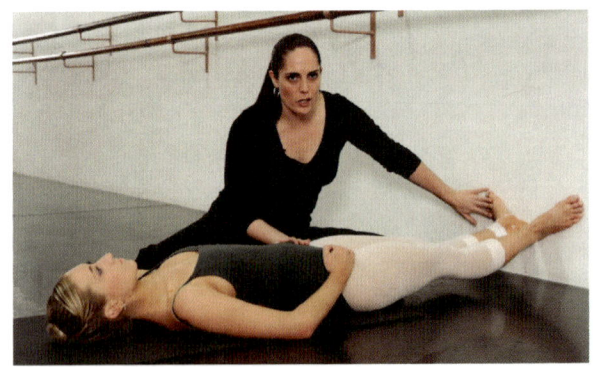

3. Slowly turn your feet into 1st position using your deep turnout muscles only. Check that you are keeping your bigger gluteal muscles relaxed.

4. Hold for 5 seconds in 1st position, breathing normally, focusing on maintaining your maximum turnout range. Return slowly to parallel. Repeat 10 times.

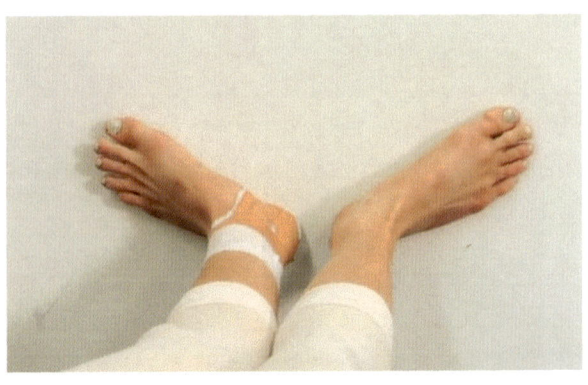

5. Ensure that you don't try to screw your feet against the wall to increase your turnout as this can cause increased loading through your knees and ankles.

Will I Ever DANCE Again?

Floor Barre - Plié

The first exercise in class is usually a plié exercise, and just like a plié in class this floor barre exercise requires you to activate your deep turnout muscles whilst maintaing core activation. Some dancers find that their lower back tends to arch as they draw their legs in, so be sure to keep your deep abdominals working throughout. A floor barre plié involves moving the legs away from the wall so I recommend that you wear some socks to allow your feet to move smoothly on the floor.

1. Start with your feet on the wall in parallel then slowly rotate feet into 1st position, maintaining neutral spine with deep abdominals activated.

2. Move slowly into a demi plié by drawing the feet halfway up towards your buttocks, rotating deeply from the hips to use your full turnout.

3. Push through the heels, maintaining your turnout as you straighten your legs to place the feet back onto the wall. Repeat a second time to the demi plié position.

4. Once you feel comfortable with a demi plié, try moving into a grande plié by drawing the feet up further. Focus on using your turnout the whole way through the movement. Keep the heels slightly lifted off the floor throughout.

5. Push the feet back towards the wall again, thinking of slowly and gently drawing the inner thighs together and fully straightening the knees. You should not feel any pressure or pain in the hips with this exercise if you are correctly warmed up.

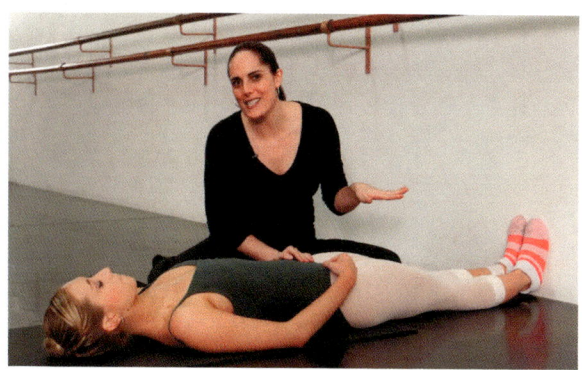

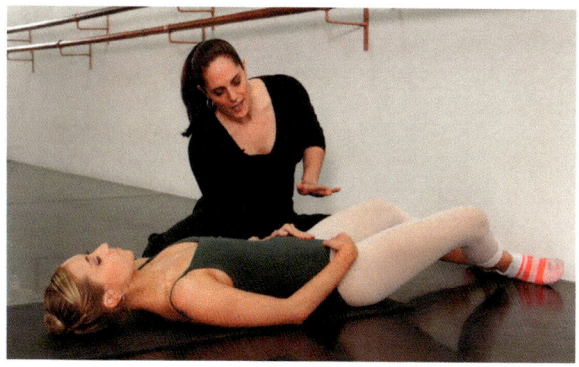

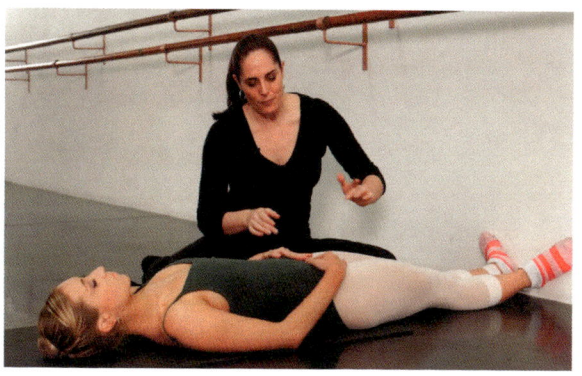

Floor Barre - Battement Tendu

> A simple battement tendu performed lying down with the feet on the wall is actually a very hard exercise to do properly. The focus of this exercise is really on maintaining control and the placement of the foot on the standing leg. As your feet are on the wall it is impossible to screw your turnout, so it is wonderful for developing true control in your standing leg turnout muscles. It also requires a lot of deep control to maintain the pelvis in a good position, so make sure to keep your finger tips on your hip bones initially to check for movement.

1. Rotate the feet out into first position. Have the feet placed in a tripod foot position with even pressure through the big toe and the little toe. Press slightly through the ball of the foot and lengthen the legs to activate the inner knee and inside thigh muscles.

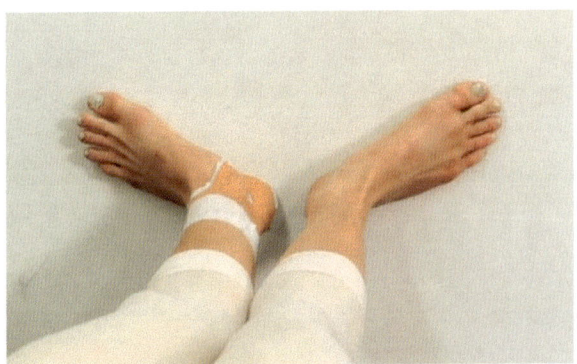

2. Push the non injured foot forward into a tendu devant, working through the ball of the foot. Make sure to lengthen through the front of the ankle and then the toes. Ensure that the toes are lengthened and not curling under.

3. Focus on the placement of the supporting leg and foot. Make sure that your hip bones are level, and that the hip of the working leg has not dropped down towards the floor.

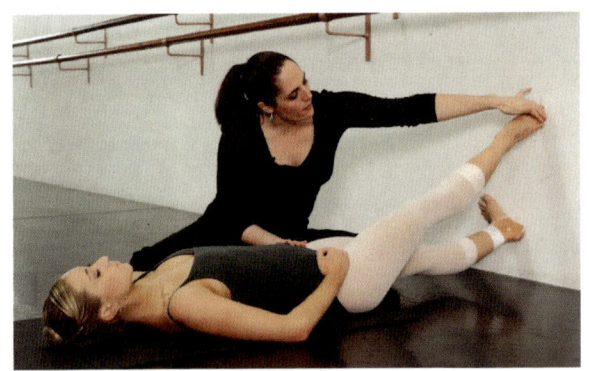

4. Slowly draw the working foot back into first position, pulling back slightly with the little toe, keeping the heel forward. This helps to work the turnout muscles at the top of the leg.

5. Keep the deep abdominals gently engaged, and the spine in neutral throughout this exercise, as though you could balance a very full glass of water on the lower abdomen and not spill it.

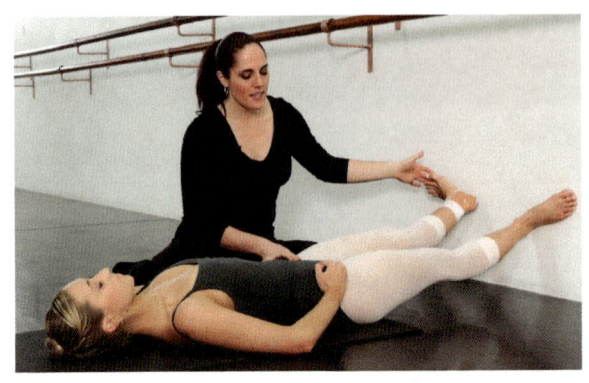

Will I Ever DANCE Again?

6. Make sure to bring the feet back to a good first position in between each battement tendu. The heel of the supporting leg may tend to drop a little if you are not effectively maintaining turnout on that side.

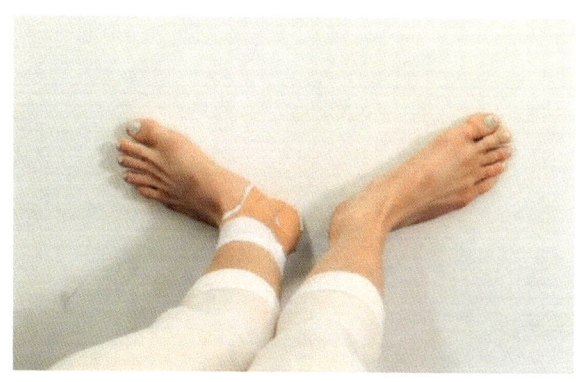

7. Perform at least four tendu devant with the non injured foot, consistently working to keep the position of the supporting leg maintained.

8. Repeat the exercise on the injured foot, taking care to follow any variations given to you by your treating health professional. If you have any problems in the back of the ankle, you may need to keep the injured foot flexed.

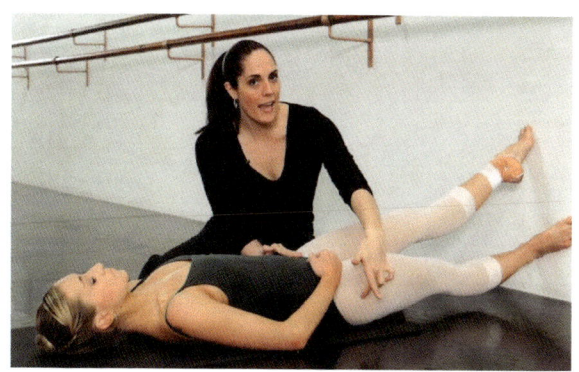

9. Repeat the exercise on the non injured side, this time to second position. As the leg is out to the side, there is more rotational load on the pelvis and you will have to work harder to keep the hips level, and supporting leg turned out. Perform 4 battement tendus at a speed that you can control, on each side.

10. You will obviously not be able to perform a battement tendu derierre in this position, however, try lying on your stomach to do this. This variation really works your core and turnout and is good if you have pain in the front of the hips.

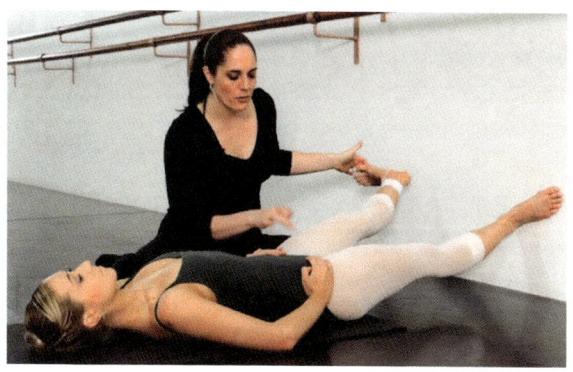

Variations: Please consult your treating health professional for the variation that is right for you. If you have an issue with the back of the ankle, (Posterior Impingement, Os Trigonum, Achilles Tendinopathy etc) you may need to keep the injured foot flexed. Other injuries may allow you to point the ankle but not the toes. If you are at the stage that you can go in a fully pointed position, make sure to lengthen the toes and smoothly articulate the foot into the pointed position.

Will I Ever DANCE Again?

Floor Barre - Battement Fondu

1. Begin as for plié with a neutral spine position. Place your hands on the front of your hips to monitor any pelvic rotation that may occur as you are doing the exercise.

2. 'Fondu' on the injured leg, by bending the knee and sliding the foot in towards your sitting bones. Keep the pinkie toe on the floor and the heel slightly lifted if possible. Draw the working foot up into a petit retiré position.

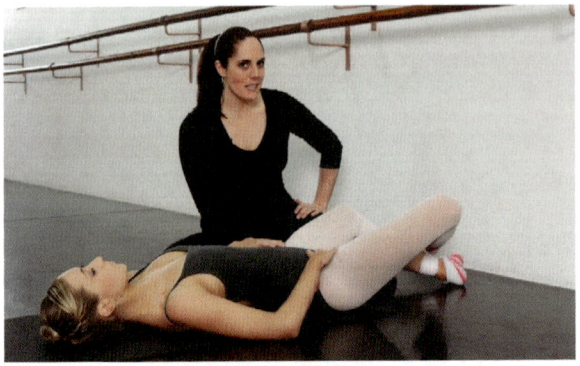

3. Unfold the working leg to the front, off the wall, and push the injured leg back to touch the wall while maintaining turnout on both sides. Ensure both knees extend at the same time, and the hip bones stay level.

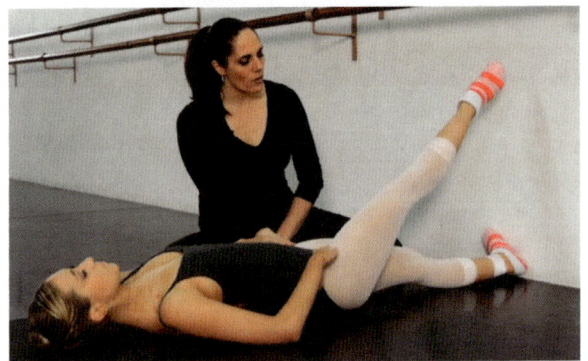

4. Bring both legs back into the 'fondu' and then unfold to second position. Repeat again in both positions. This will allow you to keep time with the rest of the class, even though you can't go to the back in this part of the floor barre.

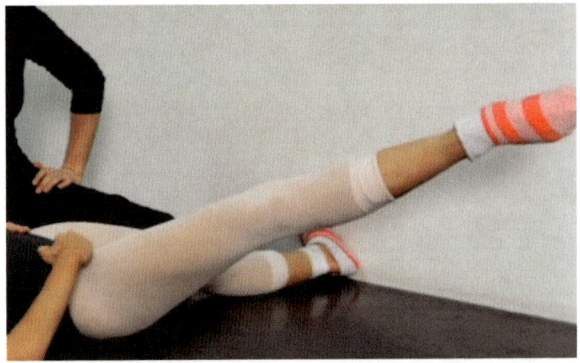

5. Repeat the exercise on the injured side when the class turns to the second side using any modifications for your particular injury. For example, you may need to keep the foot flexed, or only extend to a demi pointe position.

Variations: This exercise can also be done with boot on if the foot needs to be immobilised. Another progression would be to add in a simple port de bras, as long as you have good awareness and control of the hips.

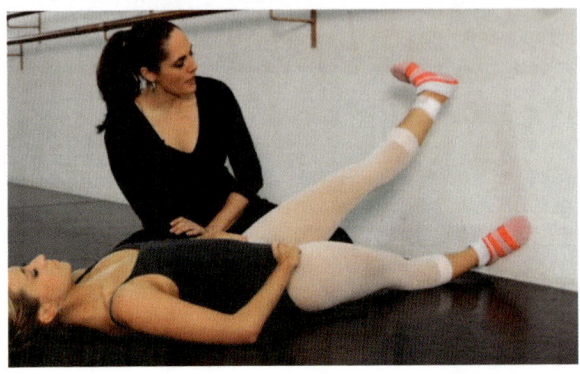

Will I Ever DANCE Again?

Floor Barre - Rond de Jambe à Terre

A simple rond de jambe à terre suddenly becomes a very challenging exercise when performed as part of a floor barre. Because you are slowly lowering the working leg to the side, the load on the supporting side is constantly changing, requiring you to adjust the level of control that is needed to keep the pelvis still at all times. This is a wonderful way to work out just how much effort is needed to stabilise the pelvis, rather than just gripping on with everything you have.

1. Start by doing a dégagé devant from 1st position, maintaining turnout control of the supporting leg and articulating through the foot of the working leg.

2. Slowly control the working leg around to second position in a slow rond de jambe à terre. Make sure that the hips remain level and the supporting leg and foot are still in a good position.

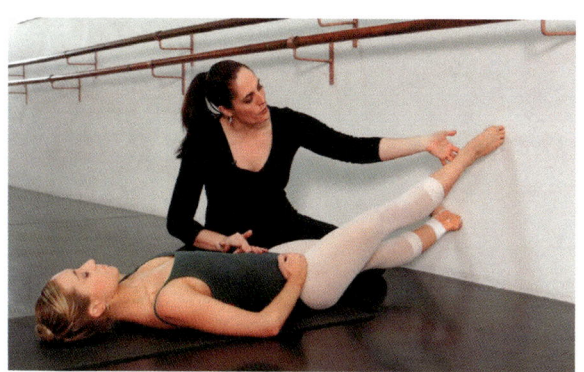

3. Slowly close the working foot into first position, working the deep inner thighs and turnout of both legs. Pause in first position to make sure that you are well placed on both feet.

5. Dégagé the same foot to second position, then slowly bring it around to the front, Check your placement before closing again in first position.

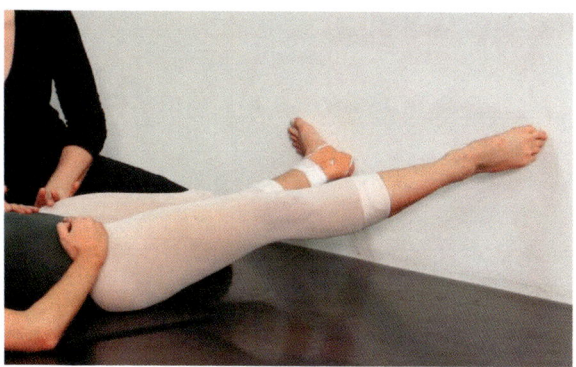

6. Repeat on the injured side with a flexed foot (or other variation). Focus on keeping equal rotation in both thigh bones throughout the entire exercise.

7. You can follow along with the class choreography, but never sacrifice your technique for speed. It is better to go at half speed to really get the value in the deep conditioning from the exercise.

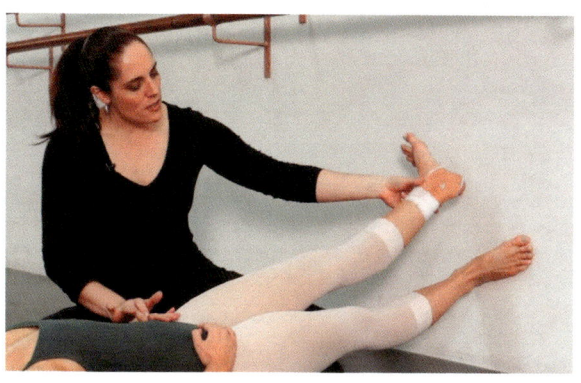

Floor Barre - Développé Devant

> Performing a développé devant in the floor barre position is a very good way to refine your technique and correct any 'cheating' habits that you have used to get the leg higher in standing. As there is less effect of gravity on the working leg, you can learn how to coordinate the correct muscles around the hip to place the leg in a good position, so that when you return to doing it in standing, it is much easier! Make sure not to flatten the low back as you take the leg devant, as this actually inhibits the deep back muscles you need to stabilise your spine. Please look at the développé sequence in the Training Turnout course for additional strengthening.

1. Lie on your back with your feet on the wall in 1st or 5th position. Ensure you have a neutral spine position. Use one hand under the low back, and one on the low abdomen to check for any movement.

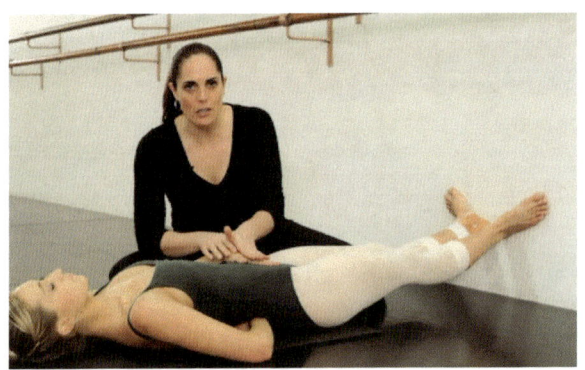

2. Draw the working leg up into a high retiré, maintaining turnout by rotating the thigh bone from the deep turnout muscles throughout the movement. Keep your hips square making sure not to hitch the hip as you bring the foot up.

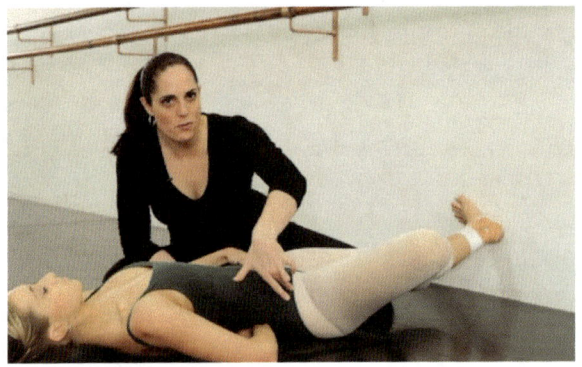

3. Slowly unfold the working leg to a développé devant at 90 degrees, taking care not to flatten the low back and to maintain turnout from the deep external rotators. Keep the shoulders relaxed.

4. Turn the leg inwards to parallel, without moving the pelvis, then use your deep turnout muscles to turn the leg out again. Repeat 3 times.

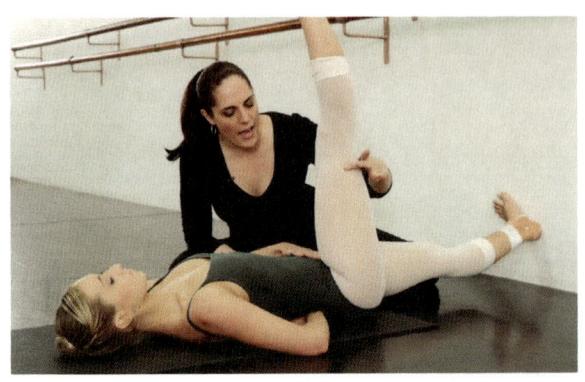

5. Slowly lower the working leg back to the wall while maintaining your turnout and the neutral spine position.

6. Repeat on the injured leg with the foot flexed if required.

Floor Barre - Grand Rond de Jambe

This exercise is a little more difficult so depending on the age and level of the student it may not be appropriate to start this exercise. However if it is an exercise being done in class then it is a very effective way of ensuring a nice stable pelvis to avoid cheating habits when performing this movement. It is a challenging exercise so it is very important to only work within a range where you can keep good alignment and control through the pelvis

1. Lie on your back with your feet in 1st position on the wall. Ensure you have a neutral spine with core activated.

2. Draw leg up into retiré/passé maintaining turnout by rotating the thigh bone outwards. Keep the hips square and stay long through the torsos as you draw the foot up.

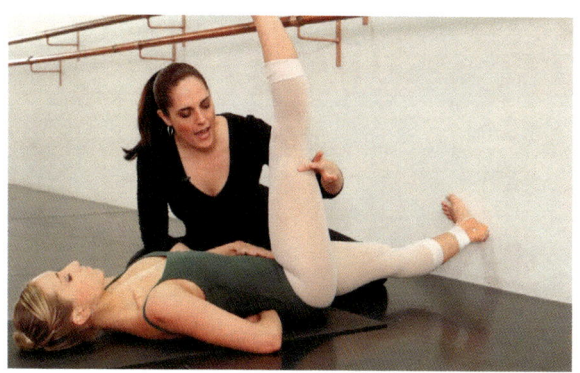

3. Unfold the working leg to développé devant, keeping the rotation through the supporting leg. Make sure you activate through the inner thighs to avoid over loading the hip flexors.

4. Slowly lower the leg out to second. Only lower the leg out as far as you can control the hips. Do not allow the hips to rotate to achieve full range.

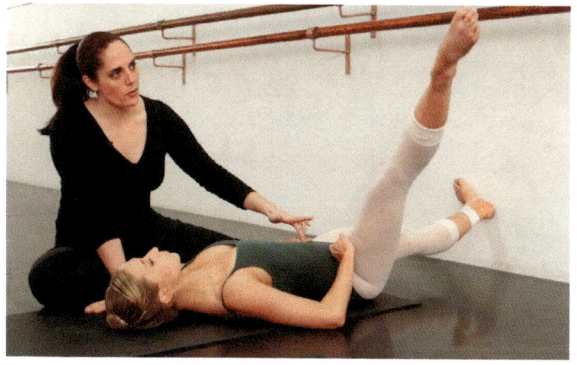

6. Using your inner thigh, draw the leg back to a vertical position then lower the foot slowly to the wall.

7. Repeat on the injured leg with the foot flexed. If you are doing this in class continue to alternate legs as the rest of the class is carrying the leg to the back or changing sides.

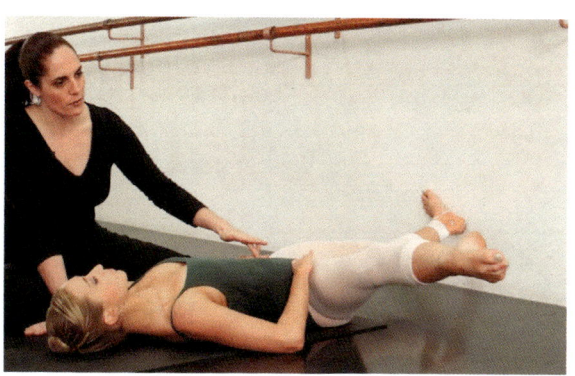

Will I Ever DANCE Again?

Floor Barre - Grand Battement

This is a great chance to strengthen your hamstrings which is something that a lot of dancers don't spend enough time doing. For this exercise you will need a medium density resistance band and somewhere to tie it that wont move for example a bed, door handle (closed door) or a stable barre. Tie a foot hole in one end of the band and make sure that the other end is securely fastened.

1. Place your heel into the foot hole of the band and lie on your back in a neutral spine position. Make sure not to place the band around your ankle. Keep one hand under your back and the other on your low abdomen to check for movement.

2. When positioning yourself on the floor, if you are less flexible in the hamstrings you will need to lie close to where you have anchored the band. If you are more flexible, you should start with your working leg at 90 degrees and only move further out if you are able to maintain your pelvic stability during the exercise.

3. Begin in parallel and slowly lower your heel towards the ground against the resistance of the band whilst maintaining neutral spine.

4. Then slowly let the leg rise back up keeping the small back muscles activated so that the back doesn't flatten. Repeat 8 times before repeating in turnout.

6. Practice this exercise in devant only. Change legs when your class swaps to the other side.

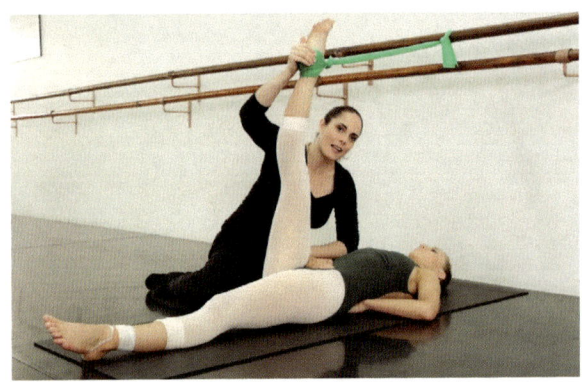

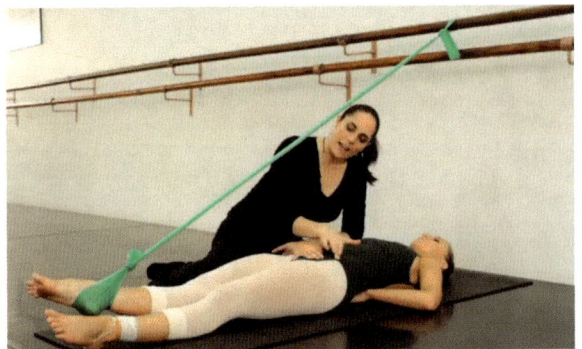

Progressions:

Try moving your body further away from the anchor point if your flexibility allows. The low back must stay in neutral throughout.

Try slowly increasing the speed of your Grand Battement, remembering to keep the pelvis and spine steady throughout.

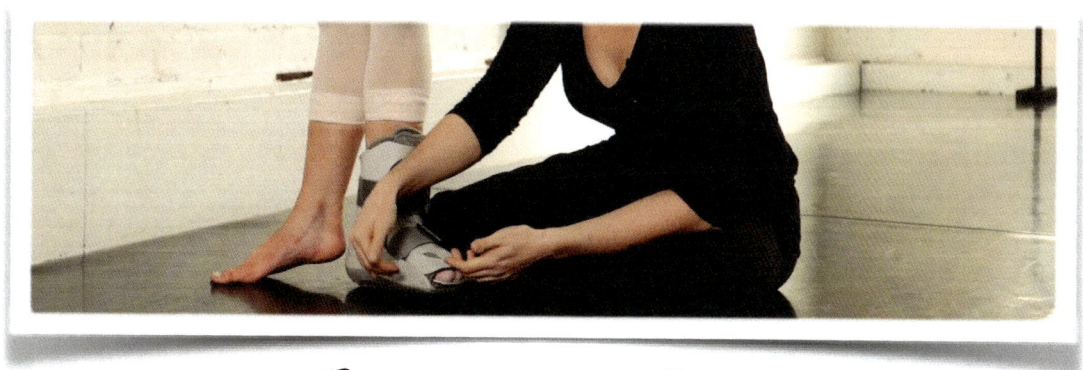

Barre in a Boot

Depending on the severity of your injury you may have to be placed in a boot. This is a frightening thought for many dancers, as they associate it with having a 'serious' injury.

Interestingly, being in a restrictive orthopaedic boot can actually help you get back into class earlier because it allows you to do more exercises in standing, without putting excessive load through the foot. However, you do need to take into account where the injury is. Whether you can do any of your barre work in a boot will always be at the discretion of your treating health professional. They can also tell you how much ankle range you are allowed to use and the Boot Barre program can then be adjusted accordingly.

For example, Shay's injury was in her mid foot so we were able to allow a small amount of movement in the ankle. Some injuries may require the ankle to be completely immobilised, so you will not be able to fondu on that side, however some barre work can still be done. Some injuries may also need to be non-weight-bearing, so you may need to continue with the floor barre, with the booted leg resting on a pillow.

Please remember that not all dancers will have the strength to be able to do these barre exercises. If you feel any overloading in the front of the hip when lifting the boot off the floor, then it is better to do a floor barre rather than the boot barre, as you do not want to develop a hip injury as well.

As the boot adds length to the leg - the other leg will be at a different height. For older students, Boot Barre exercises can be done on a mini rise while in younger students it is more advisable to wear a jazz boot or running shoe on the other foot.

Will I Ever DANCE Again?

Boot Barre - Plie

When performing plié a few variations are required in each foot position. Please watch the dvd or online videos carefully before you begin this exercise. Just like the floor barre plié, boot barre plié are a great way of maintaining deep turnout and core control. Depending on your specific injury the amount of ankle mobility and therefore the depth of plié you are allowed to do may change. In any injury you will need to keep your plié more shallow than normal so that you are not pushing on the boot too much.

1. Stand with the feet in first position, with the uninjured foot either in a mini rise position, or in a jazz shoe. It is important that the hips stay level throughout the whole plié exercise. This is definitely tiring for the supporting foot, but as long as awareness is maintained on keeping even weight across the ball of the foot, it can be a great way to build endurance.

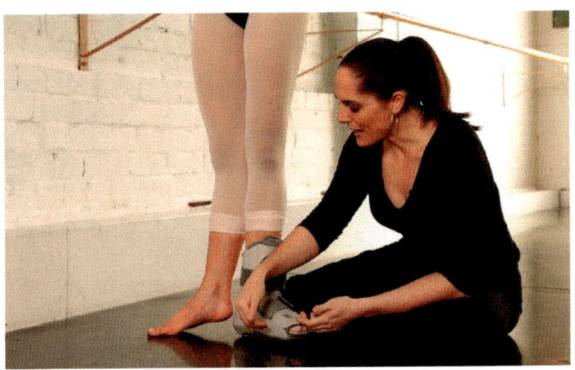

2. Do a small plié in first (more shallow then normal) depending on the guidelines given to you by your therapist. Make sure to bend both knees to the same degree.

3. Remember to activate your deep turnout muscles and draw up through the inner thighs as you straighten the knees. Perform two demi pilé with your normal arms.

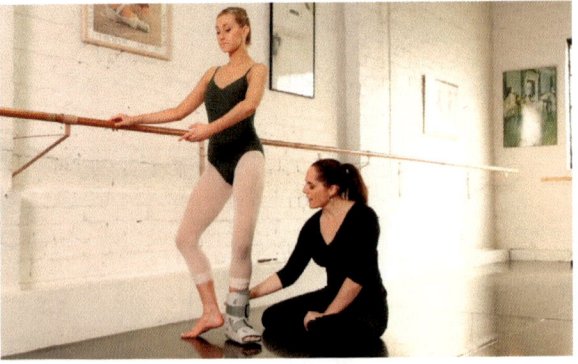

4. Perform a grand plié in first position allowing both heels to lift off the ground, keeping the hips square. Keep gently lifted through the deep low back muscles so that pelvis does not tuck under.

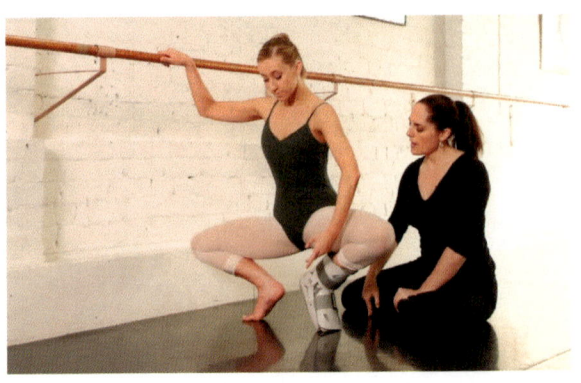

Will I Ever DANCE Again?

5. When moving into second position place the supporting foot flat on the floor. The ankle of the booted leg will remain flexed with the toes off the floor. As you move into your demi and grand plié the base of the boot will come in contact with the floor.

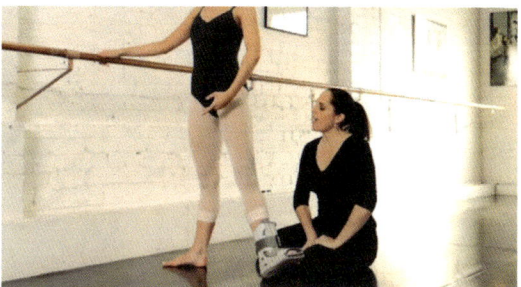 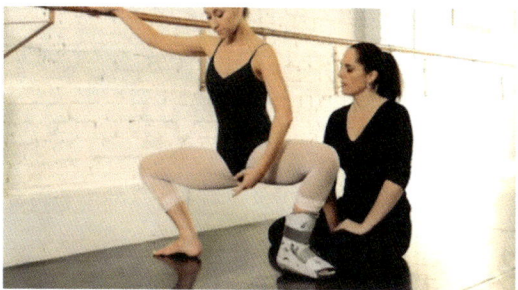

6. In fourth position, rest on the outer surface of the boot. When doing the demi plié the boot will come into full contact of the ground. Ensure that the knee does not drop forward, but is aligned over the second toe. Do not do a grand plié in fourth in the boot as it places a lot of load on the knee.

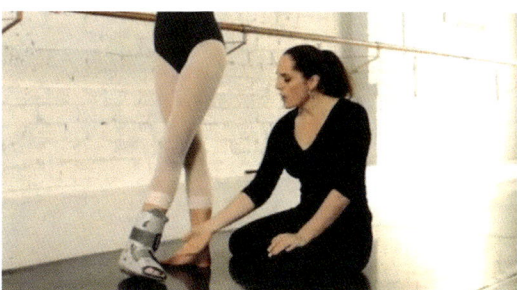 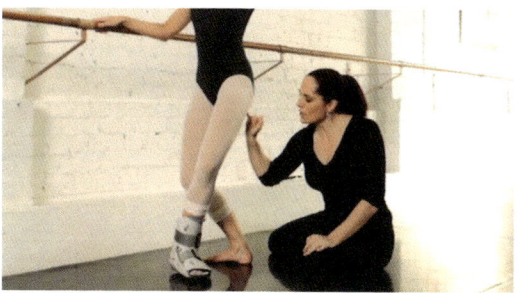

7. In fifth position with the booted foot in front, the back heel will need to remain slightly raised. Ensure there is equal weight bearing on each foot.

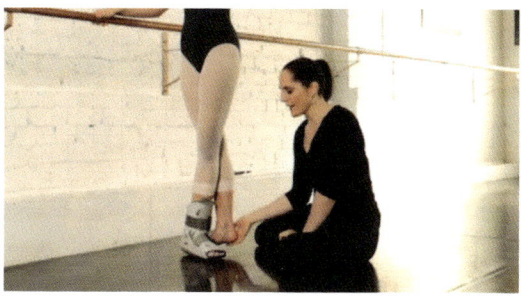 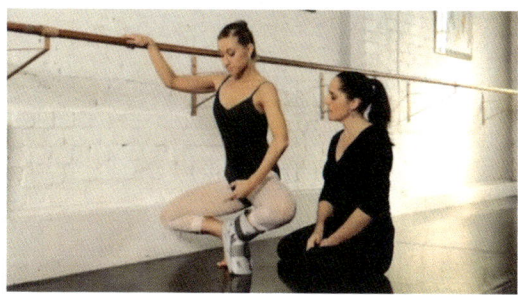

8. When having the foot with the boot closest to the barre, your plié in first position will be the same as on the other side. Think carefully about the position of your foot inside the boot and ensure you have equal weight placement between your big toe and your little toe on both feet.

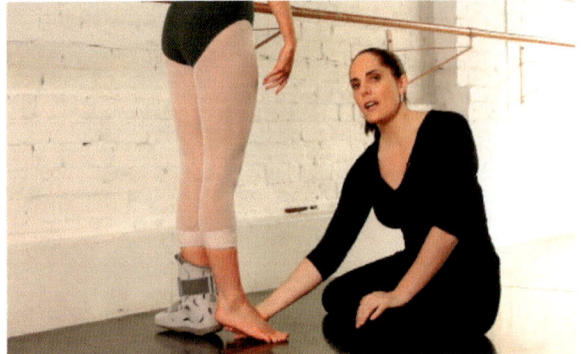

9. When doing a plié in second with the booted leg close to the barre you will need to move it under the barre a little so you can share the weight more evenly and still reach the barre. Make sure to maintain your tripod foot position on the supporting leg

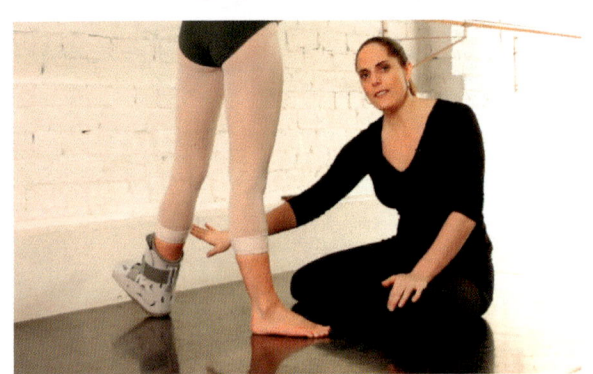

10. In fourth position start with both feet flat on the ground. Wrap your turnout muscles and perform a shallow demi plié. As you move into the demi plié your booted (back) foot will come slightly off the ground. Remember not to perform grand plies in fourth position while in the boot.

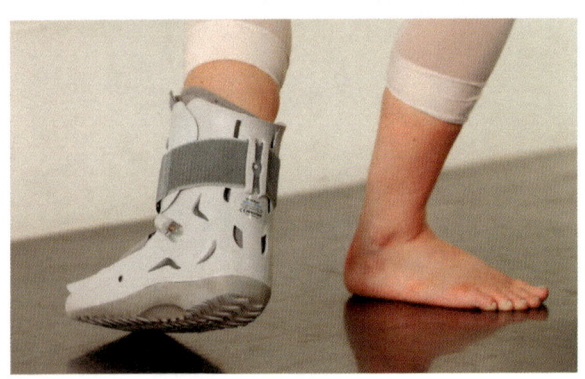

11. In fifth position keep the front (unbooted) foot on a small rise to maintain a level pelvis position. Remember to keep your demi plié quite shallow and activate your deep turnout and deep back muscles throughout your grand plié.

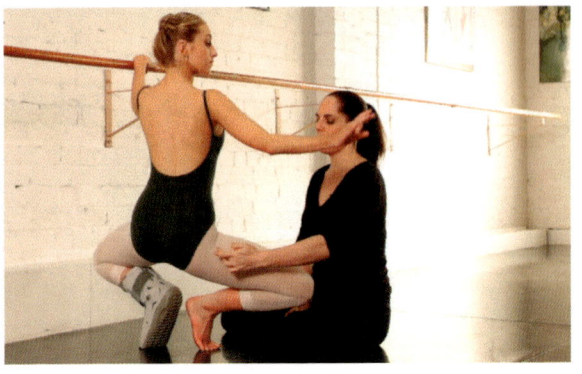

Will I Ever DANCE Again?

Boot Barre - Battement Tendu

This Battement Tendu exercises can be quite challenging depending on the age and capability of the dancer as the heel of the supporting leg needs to be slightly raised when using the booted leg as the working leg. If the supporting leg is fatiguing it is advisable to wear a jazz boot on the non-booted leg. If you are doing this exercise during class, you can try your normal set exercise as long as the music is not too fast, or you can try a simple Tendu en Croix as demonstrated here.

1. When using the booted leg as working leg accept your weight onto your back foot, releasing the booted foot to the front. Make sure to keep equal weight between the big and little toe of the back foot and keep the heel slightly raised. Keep your hips square to the front, and maintain the turnout of the supporting leg.

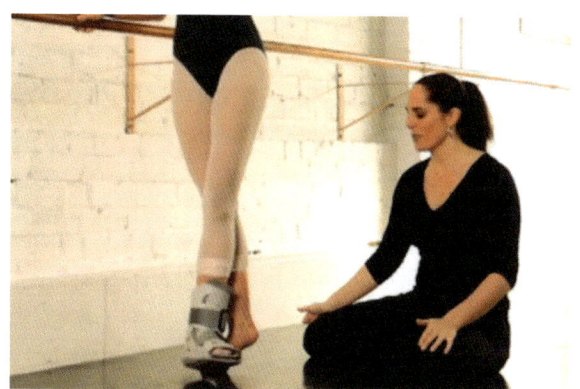

2. As you draw the booted leg back in, keep the boot slightly off the floor and maintain a mini rise on your supporting leg to allow the foot to close in fifth. For this example do two slow Tendu Devant, and then three fast ones to challenge the turnout control on both legs.

3. Repeat the Tendu to second position keeping the hips square to the front.

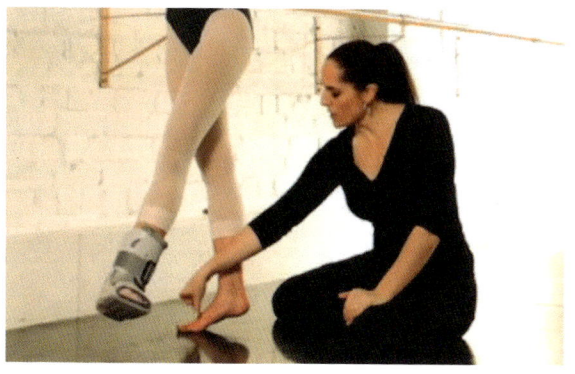

4. The Tendu Derierre is the most challenging position and many people tend to roll in on the supporting foot. Make sure you keep the little toe of the front foot in contact with the floor and maintain the turnout control of the supporting leg. Stay lifted through the front of the pelvis.

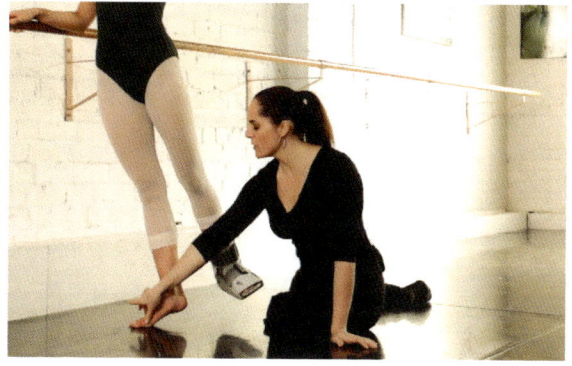

5. Repeat again to 2nd.

Will I Ever DANCE Again?

> There are a few differences when you turn to the other side and use the booted leg as the supporting leg. It is actually a little easier because you can stand on the elevated boot. Obviously if you have been wearing a shoe on the non-injured foot you can either work the Battement Tendu with it on (if it is a jazz boot) or take it off (if you are wearing runners).

6. Start with the booted leg flat on the ground and the other leg on a small rise in 5th position. Make sure to work on controlling your turnout from the top of the leg, and keep the outer bottom muscles relaxed.

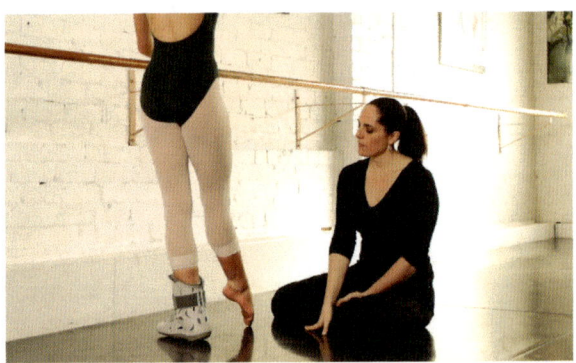

7. Slowly perform a battement tendu devant with the uninjured leg, making sure you work through the demi point and keep your toes long at the end of the movement. Do two slow tendu devant, then three fast ones, working on a clean closure each time.

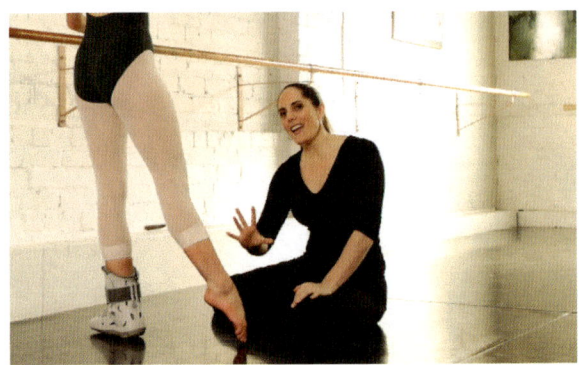

8. Try working with the un-booted foot bare or with just a foot thong on so you can really feel what is happening in your foot. It is important to really articulate the toes throughout the exercise. It is possible to mask poor foot articulation when in normal ballet slippers or demi pointe shoes.

9. When working to the back in a battement tendu derrière make sure to keep the working leg in behind you, as many dancers have it too wide.

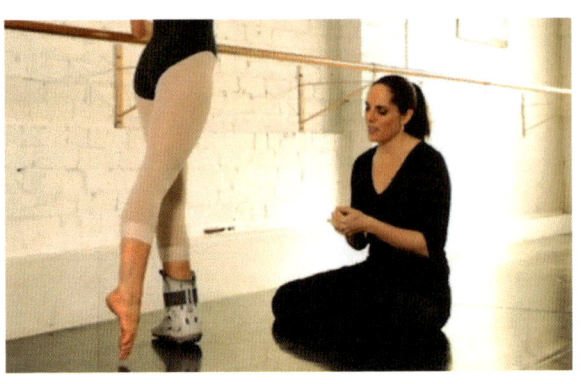

10. Continue to focus on the weight placement and turnout control of the standing leg throughout this exercise.

Will I Ever DANCE Again?

Boot Barre - Battement Fondu

> This exercise is a nice opportunity for the non-booted supporting leg to have a break. Because the supporting leg will be en fondu, the supporting heel can be placed on the ground for most of the exercise.

1. Prepare with the arms and then take the booted foot into a petit retiré position as you fondu on the supporting leg. The supporting foot should be in a tripod foot position with the knee bending over second toe. Activate your turnout muscles on both legs and keep the hips square to the front

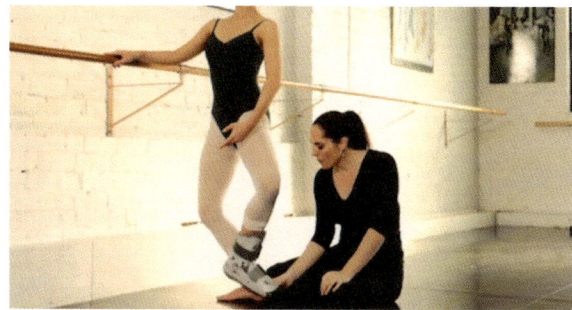

2. Unfold the booted foot to the front and ensure that both knees straighten at the same time. Repeat to the side and the back for a battement fondu en croix.

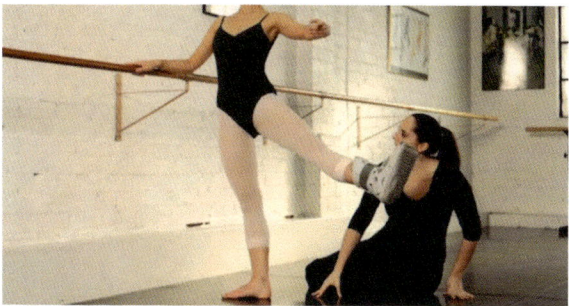

3. When taking the leg to the back, make sure that you don't pull back on the supporting leg as this can increase the tension though your shin muscles. To check your weight placement, see if you can lift the heel of your supporting leg just off the floor. If your weight is too far back you will feel that you have to shift your body weight forward before you can lift the heel.

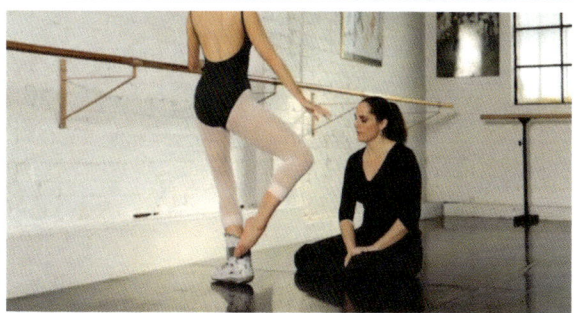

4. Do not fondu as deep (if at all) when using booted foot as supporting leg and maintain the tripod foot position. Make sure to listen to your therapist in regards to the amount of time you are allowed to spend standing on the injured foot, even when it is in a boot.

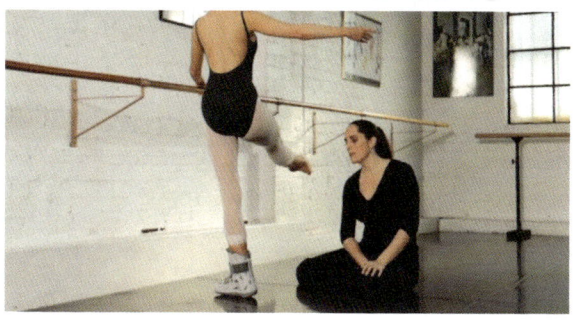

Will I Ever DANCE Again?

Boot Barre - Rond de Jambe à Terre

> For a ronde de jambe à terre, allow the heel of the supporting foot to rest on the floor for most of the exercise. When the booted leg passes through 1st position for the ronde de jambe à terre, lift the heel of the supporting foot slightly to create space for the boot to pass through.

1. Prepare by moving into a fondu, taking the booted foot devant. Keep the heel of the supporting foot on the floor and maintain turnout of both thigh bones. The more turnout you can demonstrate with the working (booted) leg, the less load there will be on the outer hip flexors.

2. Circle the booted foot around through second to the back for the first rond de jambe. As the leg passes through first, raise the heel of the supporting foot off the floor to allow the longer booted leg to pass through easily.

3. Ensure that your core is on and that the hips remain square to the front by activating your turnout evenly on both sides.

4. When using the booted foot as your supporting foot, make sure that your toes stay long as the foot passes through 1st position.

5. Some people worry that the uninjured foot will "get ahead" but this is not usually a problem. Focus on really articulating and strengthening the non-injured foot so that it is easier to 'teach' the injured foot once it is out of the boot.

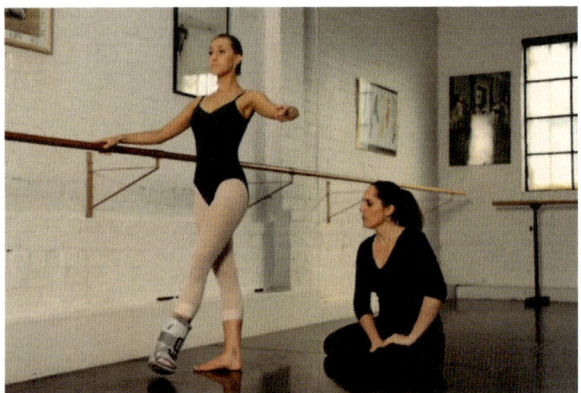

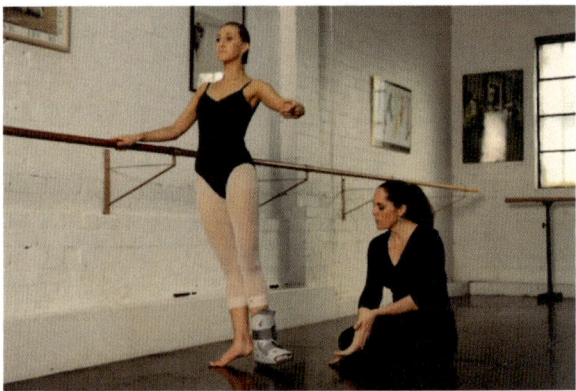

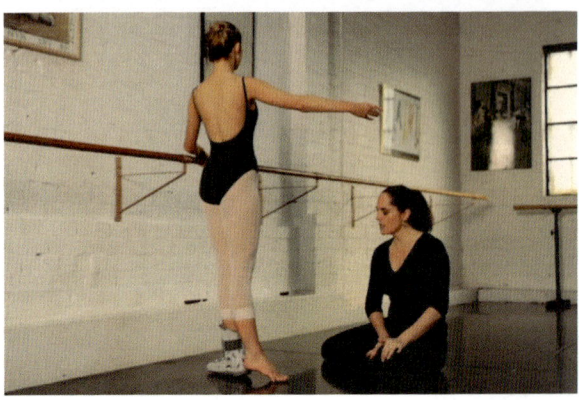

Will I Ever DANCE Again?

Boot Barre - Développé en Croix

> A développé can be difficult in a boot as there is the extra added weight of the boot when it is on the working leg. When first doing this exercise it's advisable to keep the développé at a low level (between 45 and 90 degrees) and focus on keeping the hips square, your core switched on, the supporting foot working and the deep turnout muscles engaged on both legs.

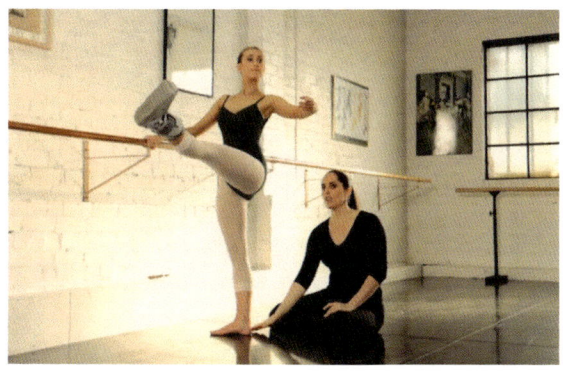

1. Start with a développé devant with the booted foot. Transfer your weight onto the supporting leg, and draw the foot into a retiré. Make sure not to hitch the hip of the working leg or tuck the pelvis under. Unfold the leg to the front, displaying the heel upward and taking care not to drop your weight into the supporting heel.

3. Lower the leg slowly, consistently working the turnout of both legs.

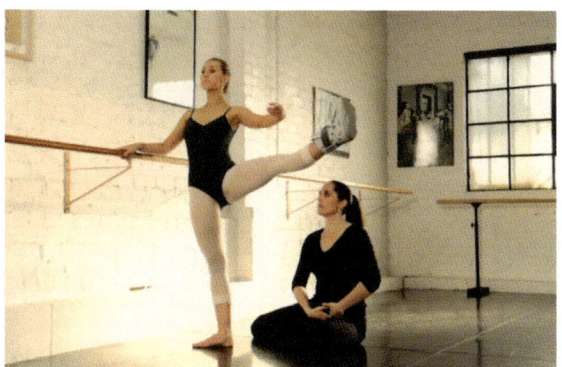

4. Repeat with a développé a la second, remembering to work your turnout and maintain the lift through the pelvic floor to support the leg en l'air. Only take the leg as high as you can comfortably control good alignment of the hip.

5. For a développé derrieré, make sure to keep lifted through the front of the pelvis to stop the hips from tilting too far forward. Work to keep the lifted leg fully rotated in the socket, and behind you.

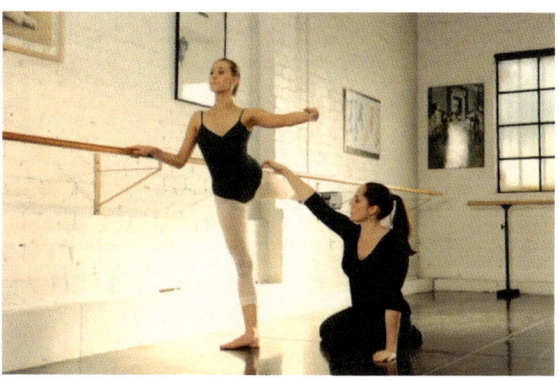

4. Doing the développé on the other side will be slightly easier as you have a stable base of support and no extra weight to lift. Focus on maintaining equal turnout on both sides and correct placement of the supporting foot.

Will I Ever DANCE Again?

Boot Barre - Grand Rond de Jambe

It's recommended to do the grand rond de jambe en l'air at 45 degree height to begin with as the added weight of the boot can make this exercise difficult. It is much better to do this exercise at a lower height rather then lifting the leg and hitching the hip.

1. Petit développé the booted foot to the front, making sure that the supporting foot is placed in the tripod foot position and the supporting leg turnout is working. Keep the leg at 45 to 90 degrees depending the level of the student.

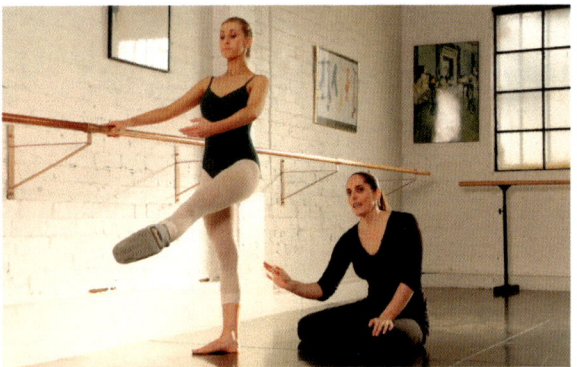

2. Perform a grand rond de jambe en l'air with the booted foot. Take special care when moving through second to derrière, making sure not to allow the hip of the working leg to swing open. Instead, lift up through the front of the pelvis, and keep the working hip pulling forward a little as the leg moves through to the position in derrière.

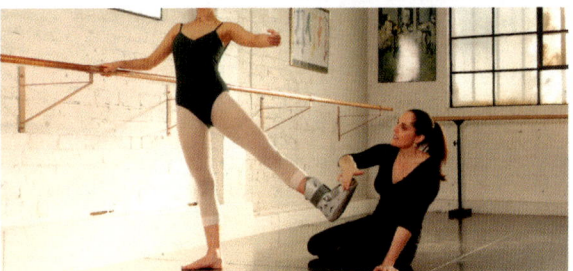

3. Keep the leg fully rotated in the socket and use the inner thighs and medial hamstrings to bring it fully into line. Close the booted foot behind in fifth, working the turnout of both legs.

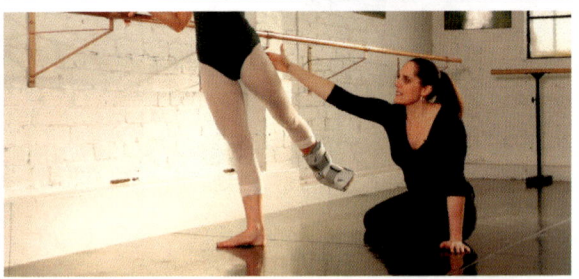

4. Repeat in reverse and really feel the hips rotating in the socket as you carry the leg around. Focus on the alignment of the pelvis at all times.

5. When the booted foot is the supporting leg, you can take the working leg to full height as long as the position of the (booted) supporting foot is maintained.

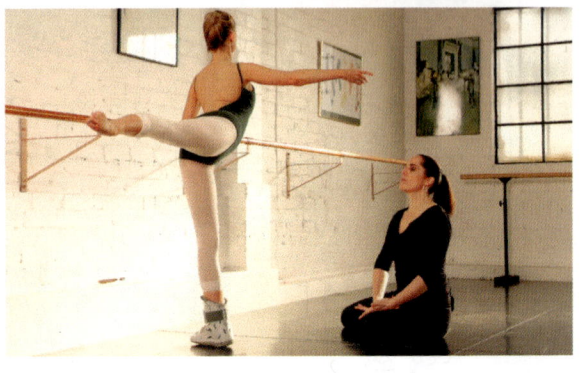

Will I Ever DANCE Again?

Boot Barre - Grand Battement

When it comes to doing a grand battement I advise that you do not to do this in the boot in standing. The sudden jerky movement of a grand battement even at the barre can actually shift the injury in the boot. Therefore when it comes to grand battement part of class I encourage you to do the Floor Barre Exercise using a resistance band or alternatively just do a grand battement in lying without the band.

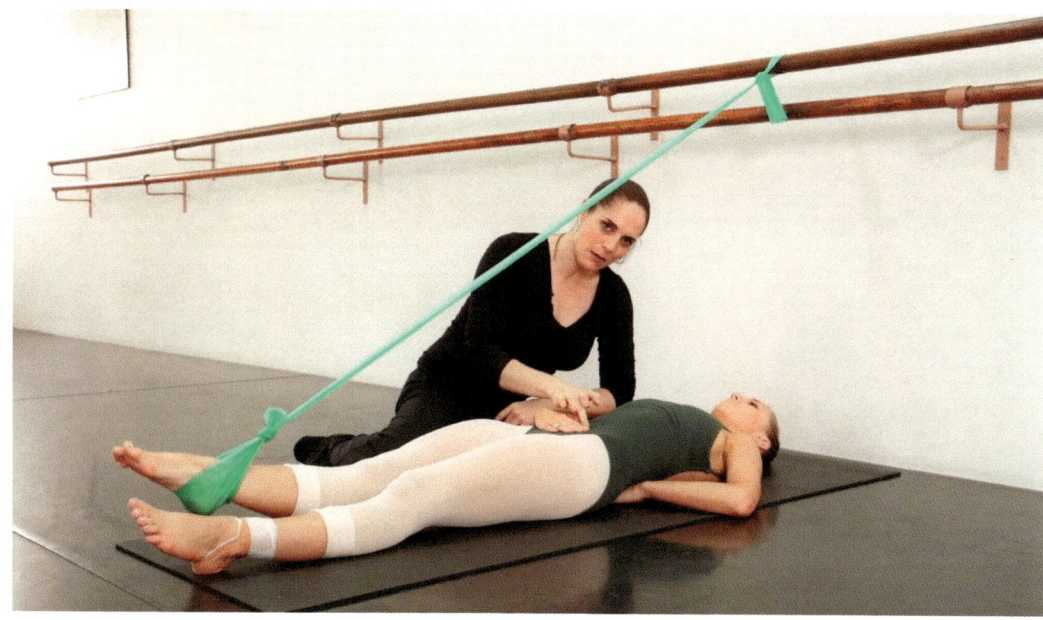

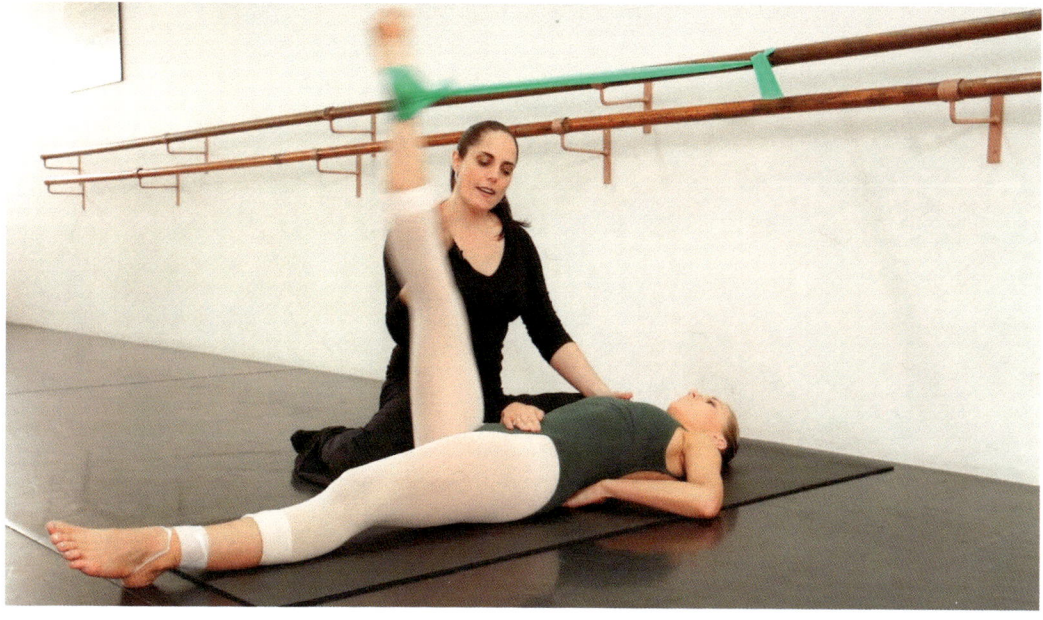

Will I Ever DANCE Again?

Will I Ever DANCE Again?

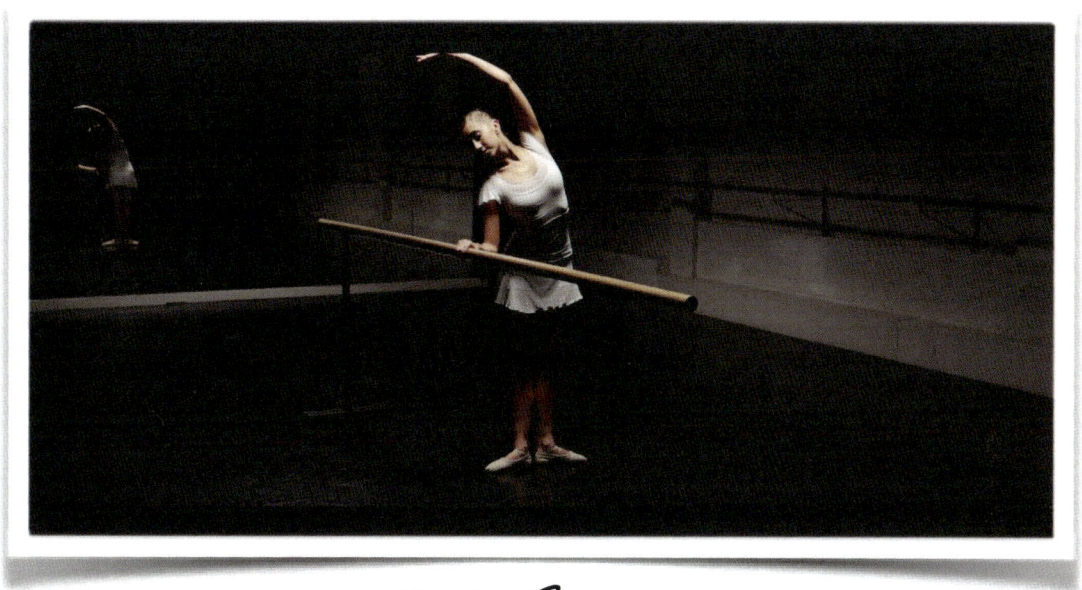

Flat Barre

When you are able to begin work in standing with the foot unsupported, you must take this gently. Often you will start work in standing even when you are not able to fully pointe the ankle. This means that you must keep the foot flexed for every tendu and développé, as well as refrain from rising.

This may initially sound like there will be nothing to do however, once you work your way slowly through the repertoire you will discover that you can actually do quite a lot of the barre work, and that keeping the foot flexed really encourages you to use your turnout.

The focus of a flat barre is to really master the control of the placement of your supporting foot in every position. It does take time to build the endurance needed to hold a good position of the foot throughout the whole of barre. In the beginning just do 2-3 exercises in standing. Gradually increase this in each lesson until your foot control can be maintained throughout the whole barre.

If the foot or any other body part fatigues, simply drop back down to doing a floor barre, rather than continue with poor technique. It is much better to practice good control in non weight-bearing than to reaffirm your rolling in standing. This is an essential stage in preventing most foot injuries from coming back.

Will I Ever DANCE Again?

Will I Ever DANCE Again?

Port de Bras

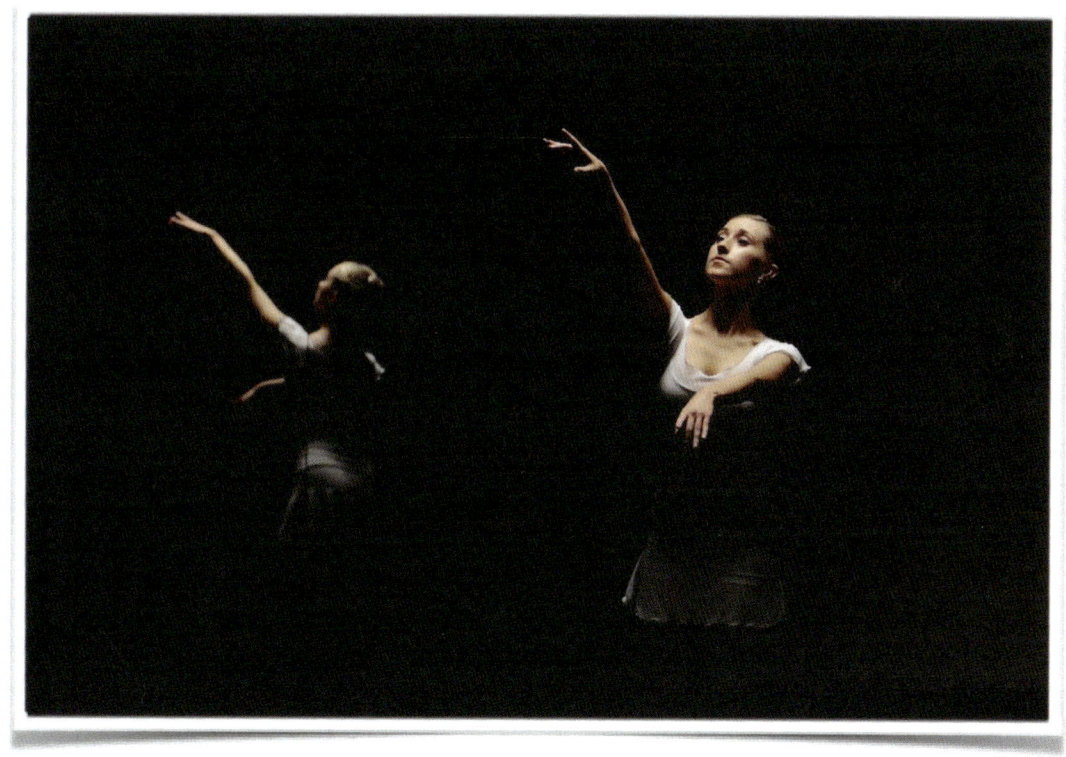

Will I Ever DANCE Again?

Will I Ever DANCE Again?

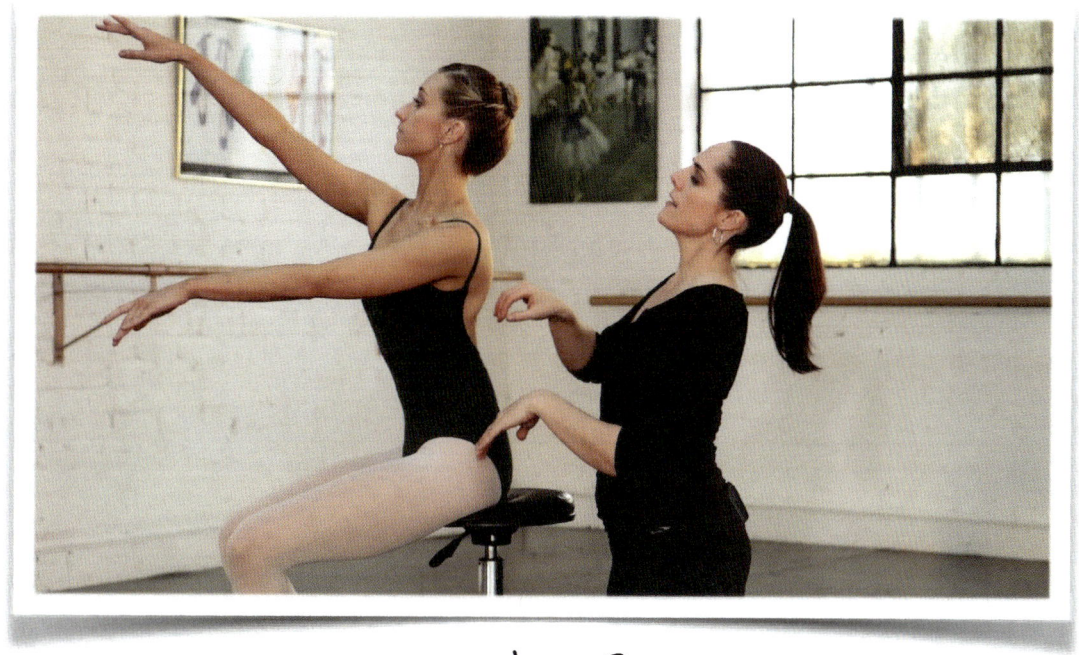

Port de Bras

When you move into the centre usually one of the first exercises is a port de bras. While technically if you are wearing a boot you could a port de bras it in standing or on flat without the boot on, it is a good chance to give the feet a little bit of a rest.

This allows you to focus on the artistry and the mobility in the upper back, which is only possible off a very stable core.

Working in a seated position is a great way to start focusing on maintaining lumbar neutral and moving the upper back off this base. Many dancers underestimate the power of the port de bra as a training exercise and of increasing their expression in a performance.

Focus on using every bone in your spine with this exercise to develop segmental control of the spine which is essential for all aspects of your classical training, including adage, turns and jumps!

Will I Ever DANCE Again?

Port de Bras - Seated

> When you move into the centre usually one of the first exercises is a port de bras. While technically if you are wearing a boot you could a port de bras it in standing or it is a good chance to give the feet a rest. This allows you to focus on the artistry and the mobility in the upper back, as well as deep control of the core.

1. Begin by establishing a good neutral spine position. Sit in a slumped position and then sit up from the base of the spine to bring the spine into neutral. Make sure that you are not over sitting and the outer muscles of the low back are soft.

2. Take the arms up into first position, focusing on softening through the chest and gazing into the hands.

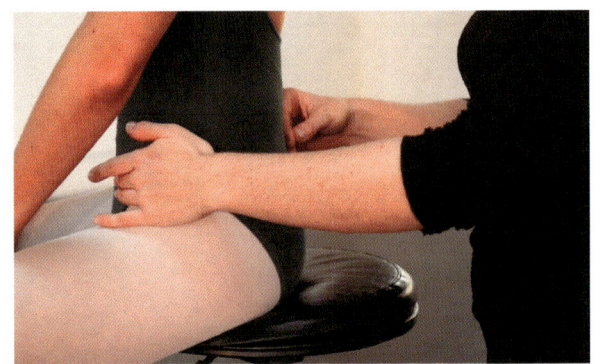

3. Open the arms out in to second position exploring how much you can expand across the chest and upper back.

4. Come into third position adding in a slight forward bend and side flexion. Look over the arm maintaining length in the neck.

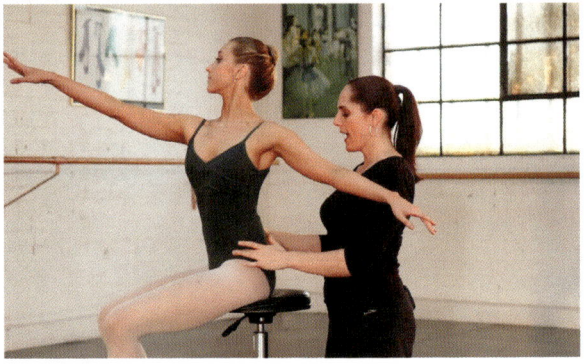

5. Explore a first, second and third arabesque keeping lifted in the low back. Focus on the epaulement, but keep the pelvis nice and stable and the back in neutral.

6. When taking the arms into fifth you can go into a small extension in the upper back, however make sure that the ribs stay down at the front.

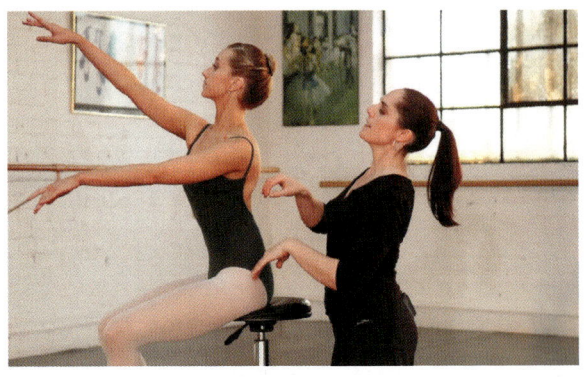

Will I Ever DANCE Again?

Adage

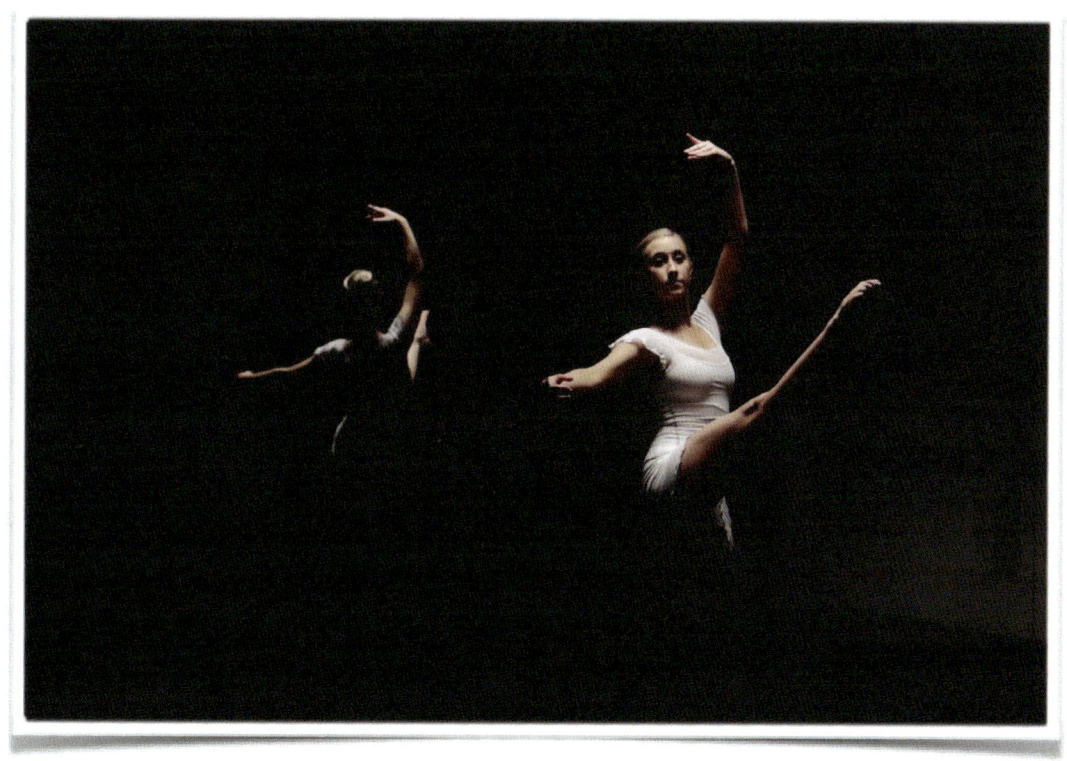

Will I Ever DANCE Again?

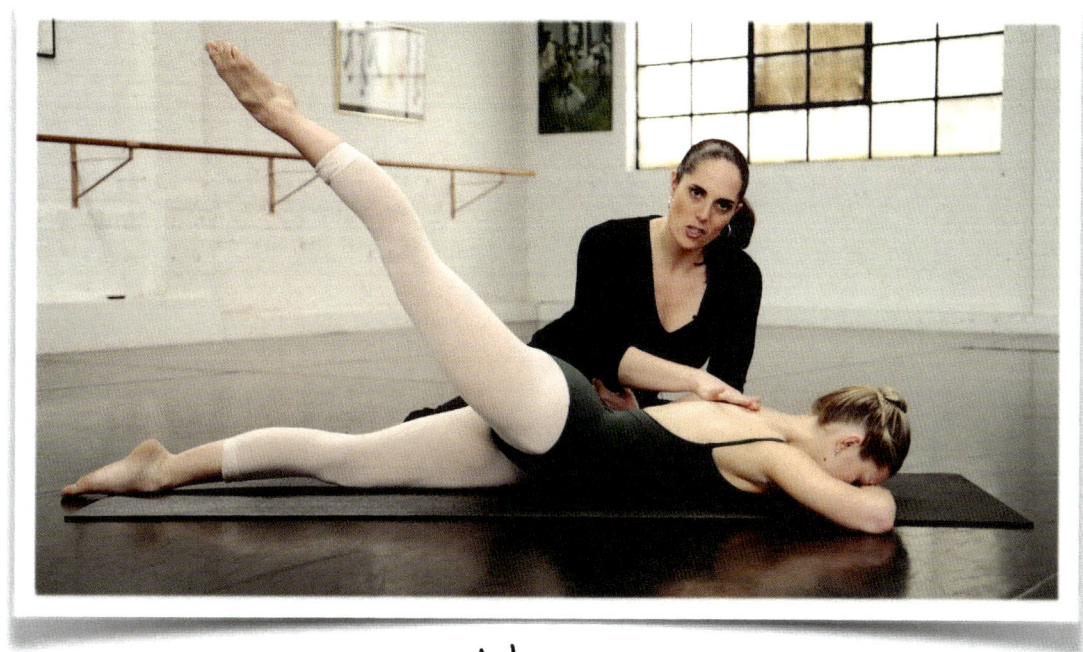

Adage

When the rest of the class starts going into the adage section of class, whether you are doing a flat barre, a barre in a boot or a non weight bearing floor barre, I encourage you to drop back down to the floor and focus on doing some conditioning exercises like the ones in this section. This is a great time to focus on specific strengthening and mobilising exercises that will actually improve your adage long term, but that you often do not have time to do in your normal training.

These exercises are all designed to develop your strength and control around the core and pelvis, as well as mobility and control of the upper back, this will allow you to achieve much higher extensions when you do get back into standing.

You may also add in any of the more advanced sequences of exercises for développé devant, développé a la second or penché sequences that are in the training turnout program.

When you are able to work in standing again, make sure that you start off keeping your working leg low in order to focus on maintaining the position of the supporting foot until it regains endurance.

Will I Ever DANCE Again?

Adage - Cushion Squeezes

The first exercise we are going to do is one of my favourites. It involves using a small ball, which is a wonderful piece of equipment for any dancer, and is available on our online store. This ball can be used for many beneficial foot, turnout and core exercises, so I encourage you to get one of these. However, if you don't have one of these balls yet, you can use a pillow for this exercise.

1. Keep your feet together and place the ball between the knees. Remember to place it quite low, as it does tend to work it's way up during this exercise.

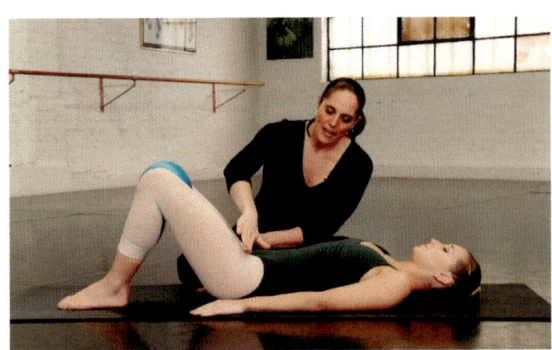

2. Place your fingertips across the top of your thighs to check that the hip flexor muscles are relaxed. This is very important, as a lot of people tend to grip excessively with these muscles when doing stability exercises. Especially if you have had issues with the hips clicking, or getting very tight, this may be a challenging exercise for you.

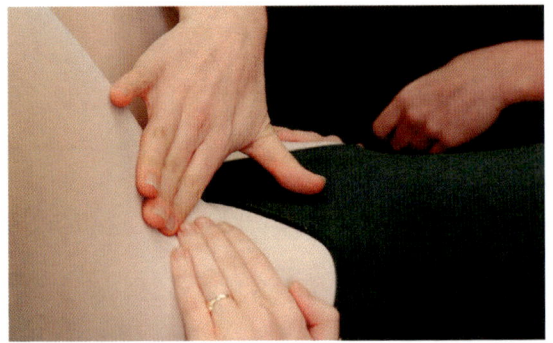

3. Make sure you are in neutral spine with a gentle lift through the base of the spine, and a gentle drawing in and hollowing of the low pelvis, without flattening the back. Keep the shoulders nicely open and relaxed.

4. Squeeze the ball, but focus on bringing the thighs together in parallel, rather than squeezing from the knees.

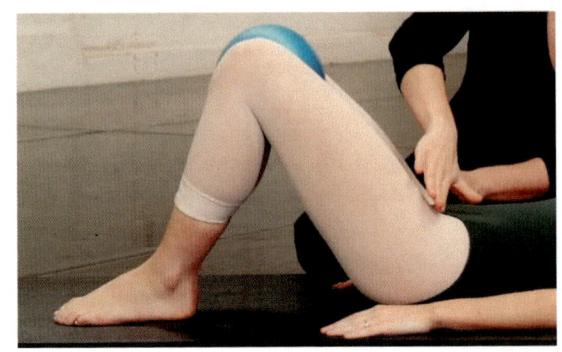

5. Hold for about three breaths, checking to see that you are relaxed across the front of the hips. Then slowly release the inside thighs, but maintain pelvic floor control. If you feel the inside thighs start to tremble a little, this is okay. You are just using the deep stabilising muscles in a way they probably have not worked before!

Will I Ever DANCE Again?

Cushion Squeezes with Leg Extension

If you can do the first variation of this exercise keeping the front of both hips relaxed, you can move on to the advanced stage. Please note that it is ok to feel the front of the working hip come on in this exercise. You cannot keep it fully relaxed, as the quadriceps need to activate to extend the knee. However do try to still keep the supporting side relaxed at the front of the hip.

1. Squeeze the inside thighs as for the first exercise and then straighten one leg, maintaining the squeeze of the ball with the deep inside thighs.

2. Slowly rotate the thigh bone in the socket, and you will feel the tension move from the inner thigh of the working leg around into the turnout muscles.

3. Rotate the leg back into parallel, and then replace the foot down onto the mat.

4. Maintain the squeeze, and then extend the opposite leg to repeat on the other side. Turnout, then bring the leg back into parallel, keeping the inner thighs gently squeezing, and then replace the foot down to the mat.

5. Slowly release the inner thigh contraction, but try to maintain the deep back and pelvic floor control, rather than relaxing everything.

NB: When you go to turn the working leg out, make sure that you do not twist the pelvis. Your hips must stay square and straight, with the pelvis and spine in neutral.

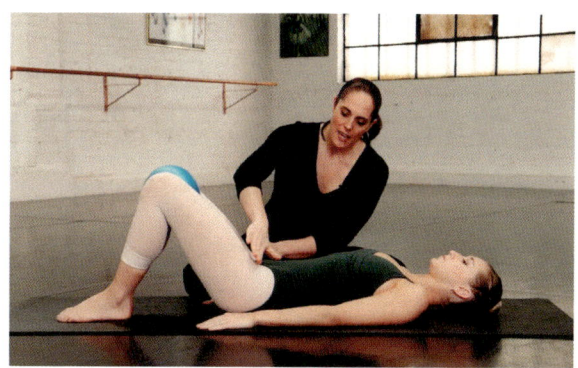
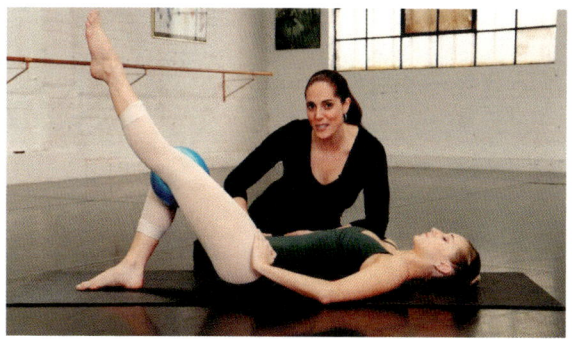
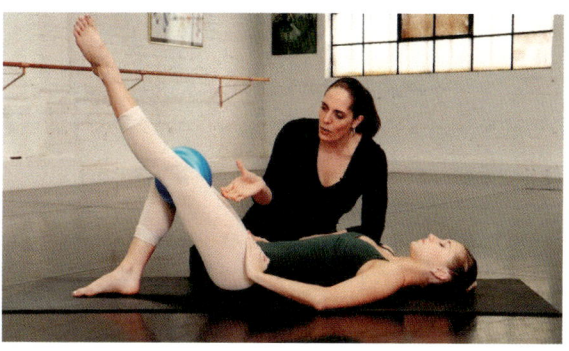

Will I Ever DANCE Again?

Adage - Full Range Crunches & Twists

This next exercise helps to improve the mobility of the upper back as well as controlling the abdominals in a small amount of extension. This is where you need it for any back bends, but this also frees up the upper back to allow the leg to be taken up into an arabesque. This one area that does tend to get a little bit stiff when you rehabilitating from an injury and are not moving around so much in class.

1. Lie with your upper back resting over your foam roller. Alternatively you could use a rolled up towel, or a small stability ball. Try to keep the roller as still as possible during the exercise,

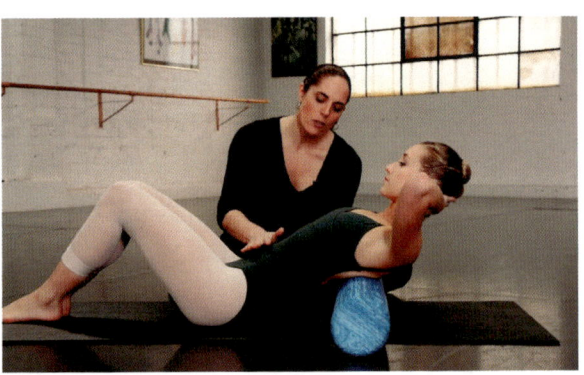

2. To perform a simple crunch, slowly extend the upper back over the roller. Focus on keeping the neck nice and long and the low back in neutral.

3. Slowly come up into a crunch up by feeling like you are bringing your ribs towards your hip bones, curling the upper back forward. Keep open through the chest area and maintain neutral spine.

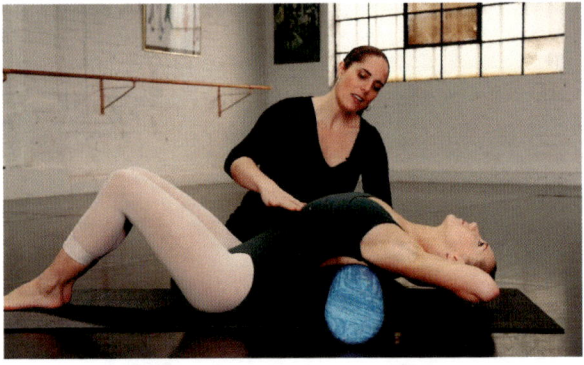

4. Recline slowly back over the roller letting the abdominals slowly release to strengthen your control into your back bend. Keep the neck long and the chin slightly drawn in.

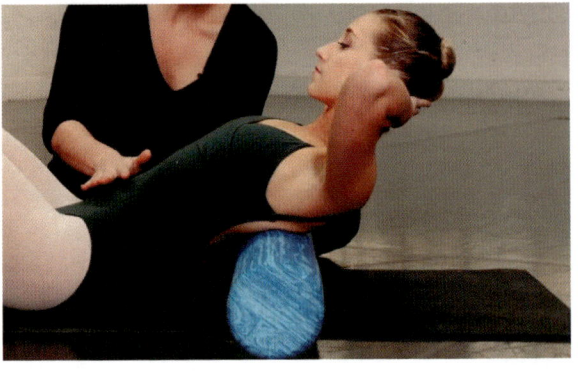

NB: You do not need to do too many of these. It is better to do a few with good form rather that lots of incorrect ones. Start with just 5 or 6 repetitions in the beginning but build up to around 20 slow repetitions once you are feeling stronger.

Will I Ever DANCE Again?

Once you have completed the crunches, you can try this variation which is a different exercise for the upper back. You may feel quite tight in the upper when you first start doing this exercise, however once you get used to it it is a beautiful stretch to free up the upper back and rib area. You actually need to have quite a bit of extension and rotation mobility to allow a full height of arabesque or attitude.

1. Relax back over the roller. Lengthen out through the back of the neck, taking care not to let the chin jut forward, and relax the elbows out to touch the floor. You may wish to place a pillow under your head to keep it a little off the floor so that you can relax into the stretch.

2. Keep the elbows wide as you slowly lower both knees to one side keeping the chest facing up towards the ceiling. This will create a nice rotation in the back, and a stretch up towards the bra line area.

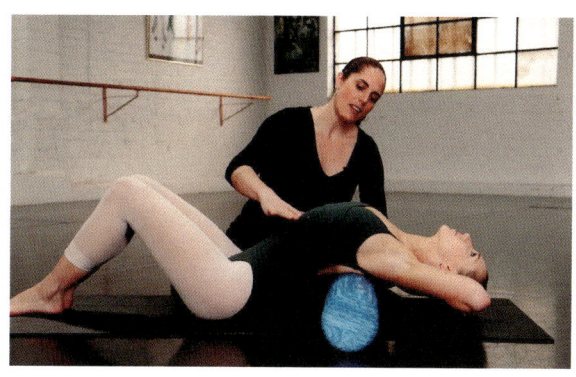

3. Slowly bring the knees back to the centre, maintaining neutral spine and then repeat to the other side.

4. You may feel tight in the upper back when you first start doing this excise. Just go to the first point of resistance, breathe and relax into the stretch. Repeat 6 -10 times each side.

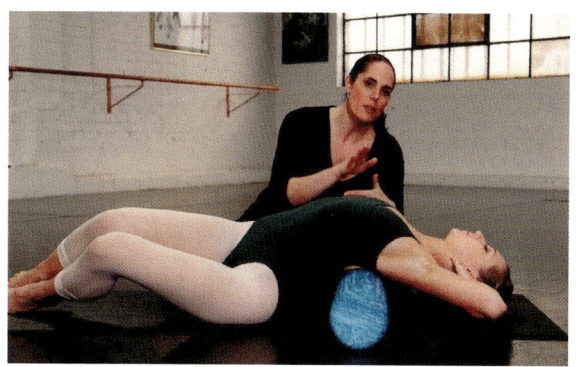

NB: If your upper back is quite stiff, you may want to start this exercise with a rolled up towel in the beginning, and then gradually progress to doing it over the roller once you have developed a little more mobility. If you feel any pain or discomfort in the shoulders in this position, this should be worked on separately before attempting this exercise. Students who have a very slumped posture can get very tight in their Pectoralis minor muscle and this can limit the amount of movement in the shoulder in this position. Please do not push into any pain or let anyone press your elbows down in this position.

Will I Ever DANCE Again?

Adage - Thoracic Sliding Version 1 & 2

> This exercise has thee variations. If you have never done this exercise before start by doing just the first variation. You can do this exercise on the floor or by using the foam roller which will make it a little bit easier to roll. If you are not using the roller take care not to push into the floor with your hands.

1. Start by resting your wrists over the top of the roller. Keep lengthened between the ears and the tip of the shoulder throughout the exercise.

2. Focus on extending the upper back gently as you roll the roller in towards you lifting the chest to face the wall in front of you. Then slowly slide back down.

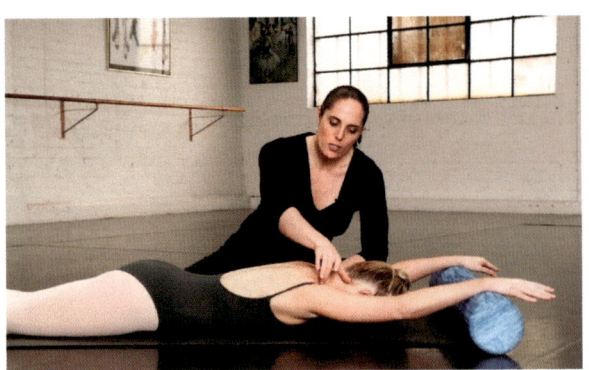

3. Remember to keep the deep abdominals on and focus on moving from the mid back rather than the lower back.

4. Keep the neck lengthened, continuing the line of the spine, rather than letting it hinge back at the neck.

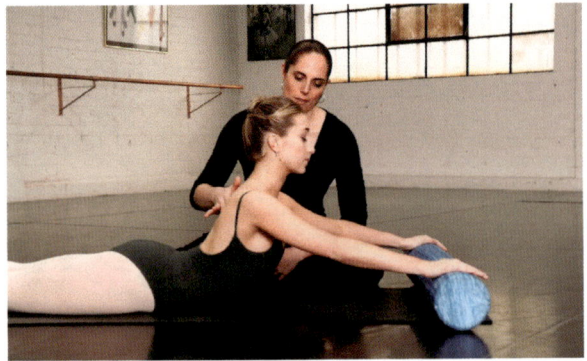

5. If this version feels okay then you can progress onto the second variation using just one arm. As you draw the roller in towards you, lift one arm up into fifth position, taking care to keep the shoulders very square.

6. Repeat on the opposite side, making sure that the shoulder blades stay wide and flat against the chest wall, and lengthen both sides of the neck. Repeat at least 3 times on each arm.

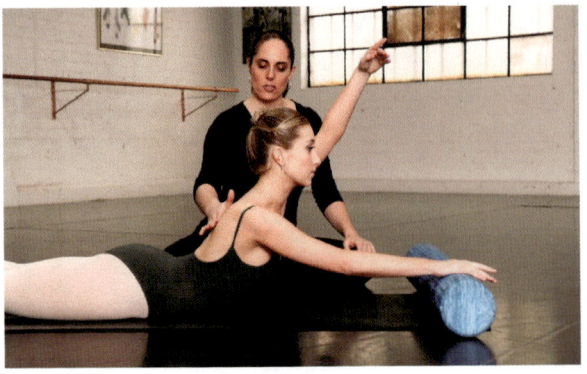

Will I Ever DANCE Again?

Thoracic Sliding Version 3

The next variation is much more difficult and is suitable for higher level students and professional dancers. In this variation we add a rotation of the spine at the top of the movement, which helps develop all the deep muscles that help support the spine when you are in a full Arabesque or a Penché.

1. Start as for variation #2 by rolling up and taking one arm to fifth. Keep the neck long, the chest square, and very little pressure on the roller.

2. Slowly roll the roller away by rotating the upper back towards the lifted arm. Keep both sides of the neck long and maintain the lift in the upper back.

3. Rotate back to the middle position coming back up to full height if you have let it drop at all, before slowly lowering the chest back down.

4. Repeat on the other side, making sure to keep your gluteals relaxed and the legs on the floor throughout the exercise. Also ensure that the low abdomen is drawing in, rather than pushing out into the floor.

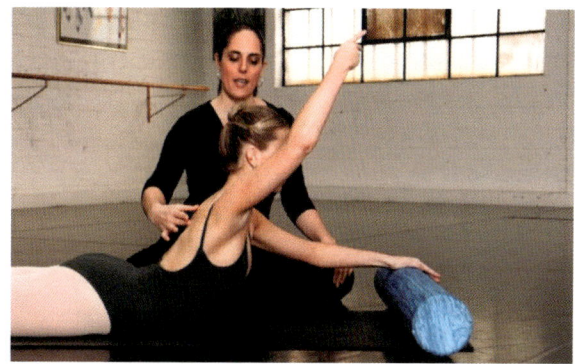

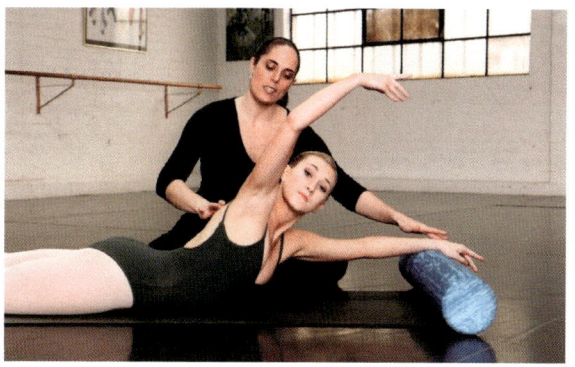

NB: You can do any combination of these three variations but please ensure that you always start with the easy one first. This is to make sure that your upper back is warmed up before moving onto the more difficult variations.

There should be no pain into the low back with any of these variations. If there is cramping or compression in any of the muscles in the low back, try the QL stretch from the Front Splits Fast Program to release it. If there is any pinching of joint pain, try a simple cat stretch and some gentle flexion or rotation exercises for the low back.

Will I Ever DANCE Again?

Adage - Stingray

This is another exercise to strengthen the upper back, which is so important to your adage, but it does it in a slightly different way. Make sure to keep the chest horizontal with the floor at all times during this exercise.

1. Start with your palms on the floor and your forehead on your hands. Keep the neck lengthened and shoulder blades wide. Activate your deep abdominals to make sure that you do not push your stomach out into the mat to create the movement.

2. Lift the upper back very slightly off the floor then side bend slowly to one side. Focus on closing down one side of the ribcage and expanding the ribs on the opposite side.

3. Come back to the middle and repeat on the other side, before returning to the centre again and lowering back down to the starting position.

4. Repeat the exercise, making sure that you do not lift the upper back up too high. The focus is on controlling the movement from the upper back, rather than from the lower back or pushing up into a big back extension.

5. Repeat 6 – 8 times depending on your strength and endurance.

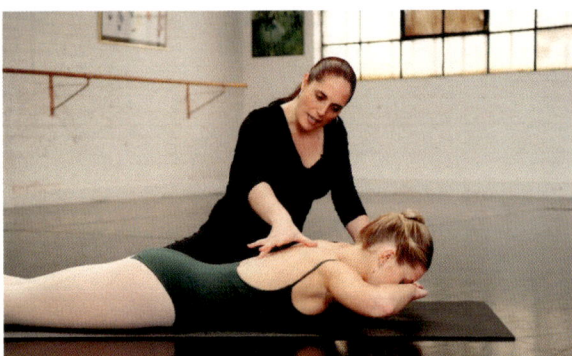
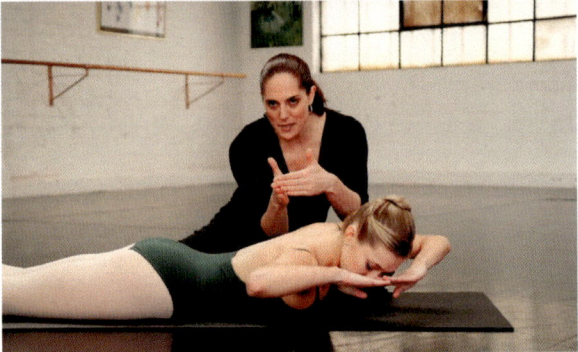
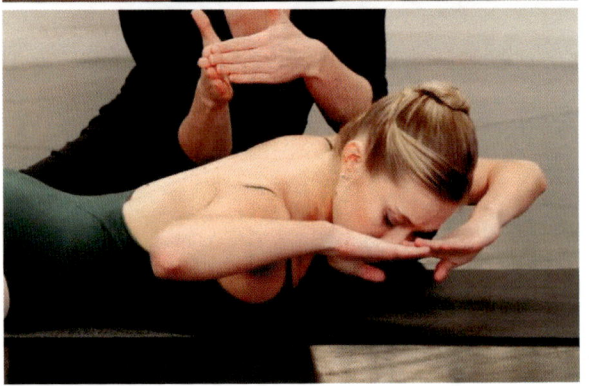

NB: Please note that there should be no pain in the low back at any point during this exercise. This exercise should be done with just a small amount of back extension so as to not put load on the lower back. Make sure to keep the deep abdominals gently activated through the exercise.

Will I Ever DANCE Again?

Adage - Retiré in Side Lying

Next we are going to start working into a retiré in preparation for a développé a la seconde. Remember to follow any restrictions your therapist has given you on pointing the foot with these exercises. For example, if you have had issues with your Achilles Tendon or surgery you may need to keep the foot flexed.

1. Lie on your side keeping your feet slightly in front of your body with both legs out straight. Lift both feet off the ground with the legs in fifth and the top leg in front.

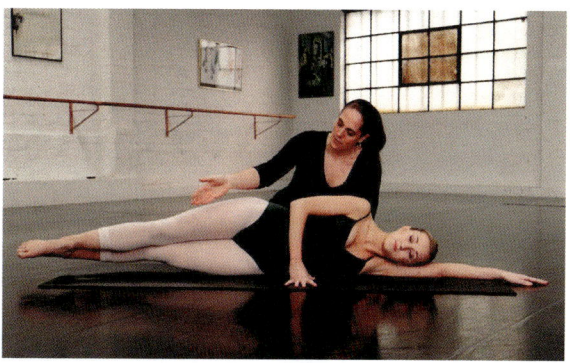

2. Gently draw the top leg up into a retiré position, maintaining turnout on both legs and keeping the waist lifted up from the floor on the underneath side. Keep the top hip aligned over the underneath hip rather than rocking backwards, as this can load the front of the hip.

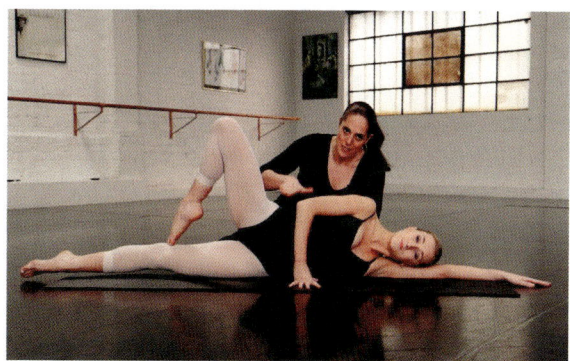

3. Slowly lower the leg back into 5th taking the top leg behind, keeping both legs lifted off the floor.

4. Repeat the retiré again, wrapping with the turnout muscles and feel the thighbone rotate in the socket. You should still be reasonably soft through the front of the hip if the turnout muscles are working correctly. Gently engage the hamstring to bend the knee, rather than hitching the hip to lift the foot.

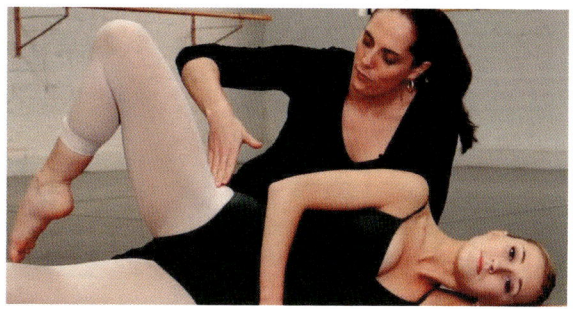

NB: If you do not have sufficient turnout range to do this exercise correctly it is better to spend your time working on this instead. Performing this exercise in a poor position may aggravate the hip flexors unnecessarily.

Will I Ever DANCE Again?

Adage - Developpé in Side Lying

> For a lot of people the retiré will be challenging enough, so make sure that you stay with that variation initially until you can perform it very well. However, once you can do the retiré more easily, and can keep everything in line for a few repetitions you can progress to doing a développé to 90 degrees.

1. Lift both legs off the floor as for the first variation. Draw up into a high retiré and then unfold the leg to a développé at 90 degrees. Make sure to keep the thigh bone pointing straight up towards the ceiling, maintaining the rotation from the hip.

2. If you are allowed to point the foot make sure to keep the toes long. Remember to make sure you follow any restrictions your therapist has given you.

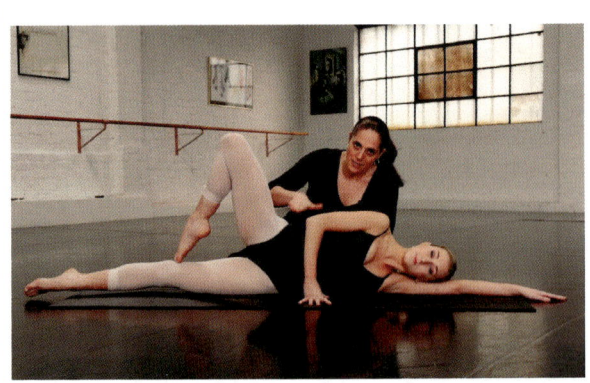

3. Slowly lower the leg to the side lift position with the top leg behind keeping the legs lifted off the ground. Repeat the développé to second and close the leg to the front before lowering the legs.

4. Once you can control this exercise at 90 degrees you can slowly start taking the leg into a higher développé, but this should never be at the expense of the alignment of the hips and spine.

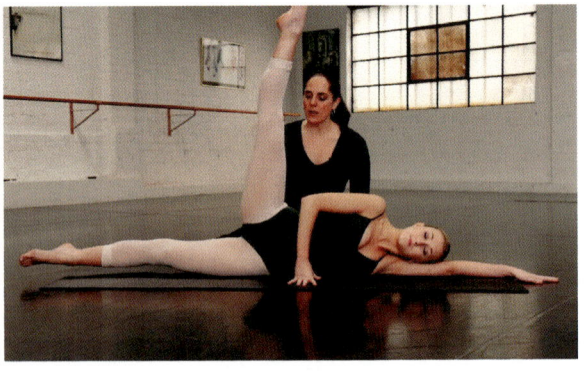

> NB: Some people find it hard to remember not to point the foot during this exercise. If your therapist has told you not to point the foot you may like to tape it in a flexed position so that you do not accidentally point it during your rehab exercises.
>
> If your hamstring mobility or turnout range restricts you from placing the leg in second position it is better to work on your mobility first. Try using exercises from **The Front Splits Fast Flexibility Program** rather than twisting the pelvis to achieve the position.

Will I Ever DANCE Again?

With Rond de Jambe en L'air

Once you have mastered the développé a la seconde you add on a ronde de jambe en l'air as an extra challenge. This should only be attempted by advanced students.

1. Développé the leg to 90 degrees and then perform a single slow ronde de jambe en l'air, focussing on keeping the thigh bone of the working leg very still.

2. If you can control this well then try a double ronde de jambe making sure to keep everything else well placed.

3. Keep your shoulders relaxed, neck long and as little pressure through the supporting hand as possible.

4. Close the working leg behind, and then repeat the développé and ronde de jambe in the opposite direction.

5. Repeat 3 - 4 times on each leg, as long as you can maintain good technique.

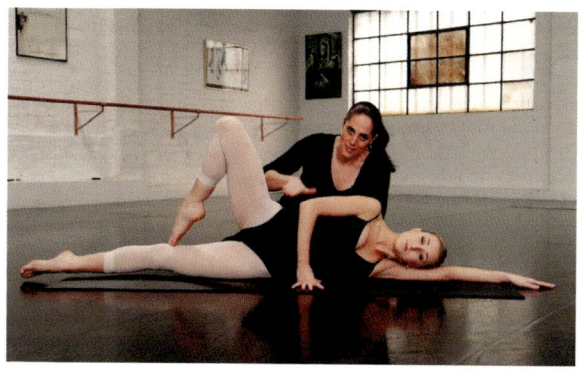

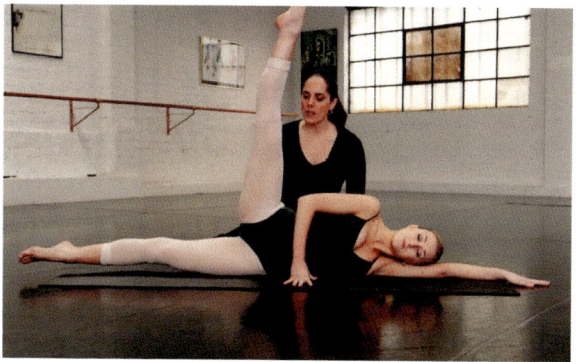

NB. Don't worry about doing to many repetitions of any of these variations initially. These exercises are more about learning how to get the subtle firing patterns working around the hip and using a little of the right muscle at the right time.

A lot of people focus on building brute strength around the hips where in actual fact beautiful adage requires great co-ordination of the deepest, smallest muscles in the hips and core. Focus on using as little muscle effort as you need, to achieve to get the desired result and you will see the most benefit.

Make sure to focus on keeping the pelvis aligned, the lower leg lifted in turnout, and the top of the hip of the working leg relaxed.

Will I Ever DANCE Again?

Adage - Parallel To Turnout

This exercise is to practice taking the leg into an arabesque without putting any load on the foot. This is ideal if you have a stress fracture or if you are recovering from surgery and are on crutches. You may need to place a pillow under your feet if you are not allowed to fully point the foot in the early stages of your rehab.

1. Start by lying on your stomach with you legs out straight in parallel. Activate the core muscles to support the back.

2. Lift one leg in parallel, flex the foot and then turn the leg out from the top of the thigh. Focus on getting the rotation from the turnout muscles and use the inner thigh to keep the leg in a good position.

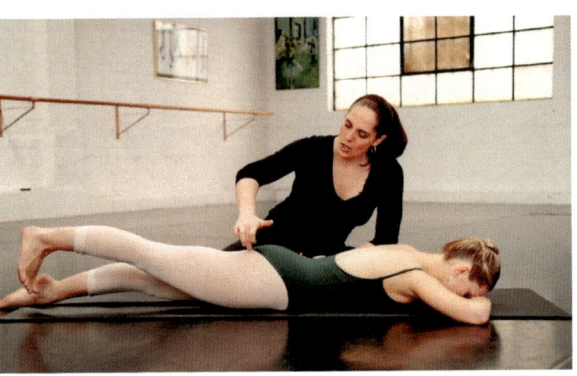

3. Pointe the foot through the demi-point position to a fully pointed position if this is allowed at your stage of rehab. Alternatively you can keep the foot fully flexed or point just to demi-point.

4. Start to slowly lift the leg higher, thinking of lengthening through the front of the hip of the working leg. Keep the leg in alignment with the rest of the body and maintain the turnout from the top of the hip. It is ok to let the hip of the working leg lift off the floor in this stage of the exercise.

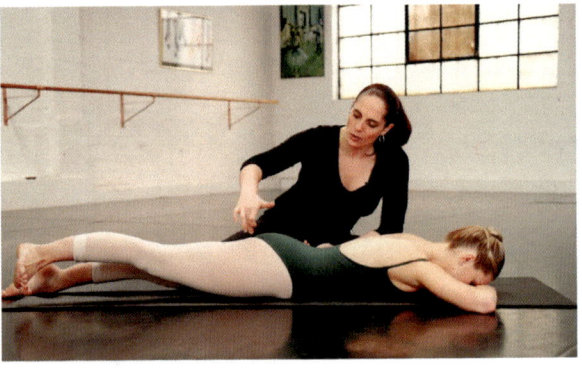

5. Make sure to keep the upper back relaxed and the chest square to the floor. Try not to press the elbows into the floor to maintain the position.

6. Slowly lower the leg back to the floor, maintaining the turnout through the leg. Repeat on the other side.

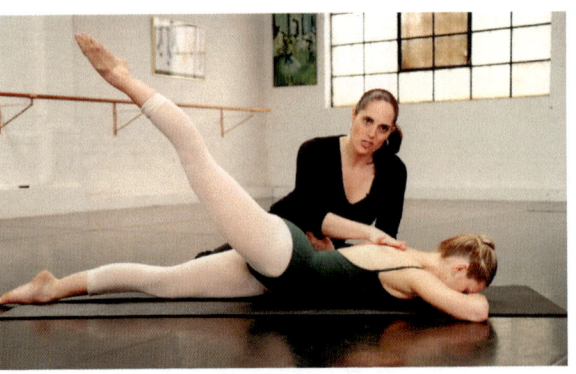

Will I Ever DANCE Again?

Adage - Building Back into Class

When you are building back to doing adage in class, especially after a foot injury it is very important to keep the legs low in the beginning. This is important in improving the endurance of the supporting foot in a good position. Retraining the endurance slowly in this way will also help prevent the injury from recurring.

1. Stand in a loose 3rd position making sure that you can maintain a tripod foot placement. This means that you are sharing even pressure between the base of the little toe, the big toe and the centre of the heel.

2. There should be a little more weight in the ball of the foot compared to the heel, as though you could rise at any stage.

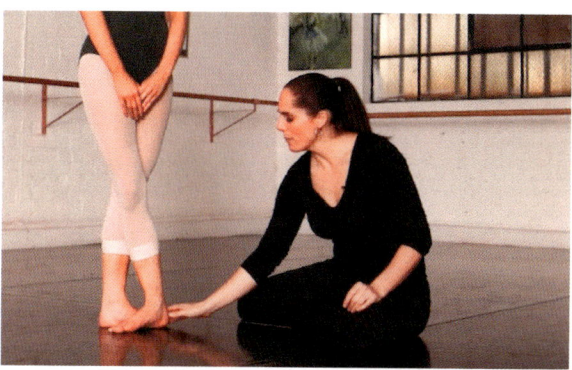

3. Peel the working leg into a petit retiré and unfold into a low développé devant. Make sure that the supporting foot is maintained in the tripod foot position.

4. Close the working leg to the front, making sure to work turnout from the top of both legs.

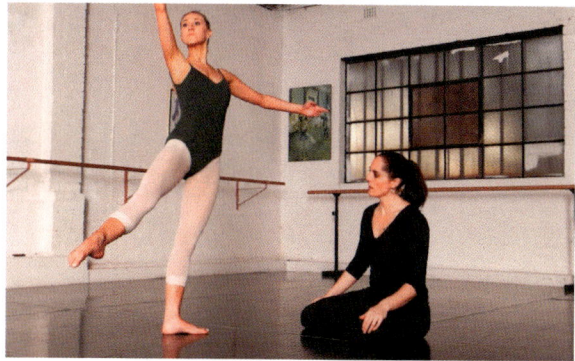

5. Repeat with a low développé a la seconde. Take care not to sink the weight back onto the heel of the supporting foot.

6. Repeat with a développé derierré, taking care not to roll the supporting foot.

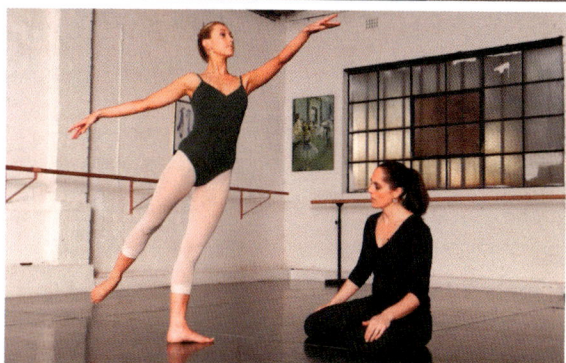

NB: You can of course do any adage enchainment that the class is working on, but take care to maintain any restrictions given to you by your therapist. Ii.e. not rising on the injured foot. Make sure that you only take the working leg to a height en l'air where you can correctly control the position of the supporting foot.

Will I Ever DANCE Again?

Pirouettes

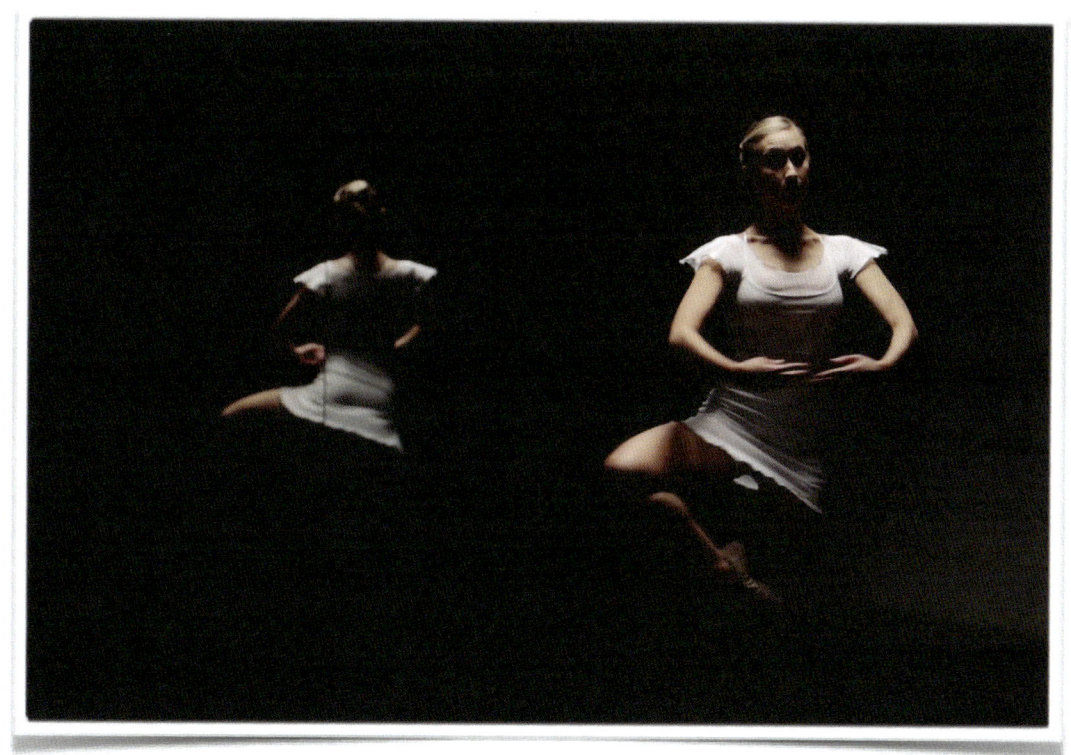

Will I Ever DANCE Again?

Will I Ever DANCE Again?

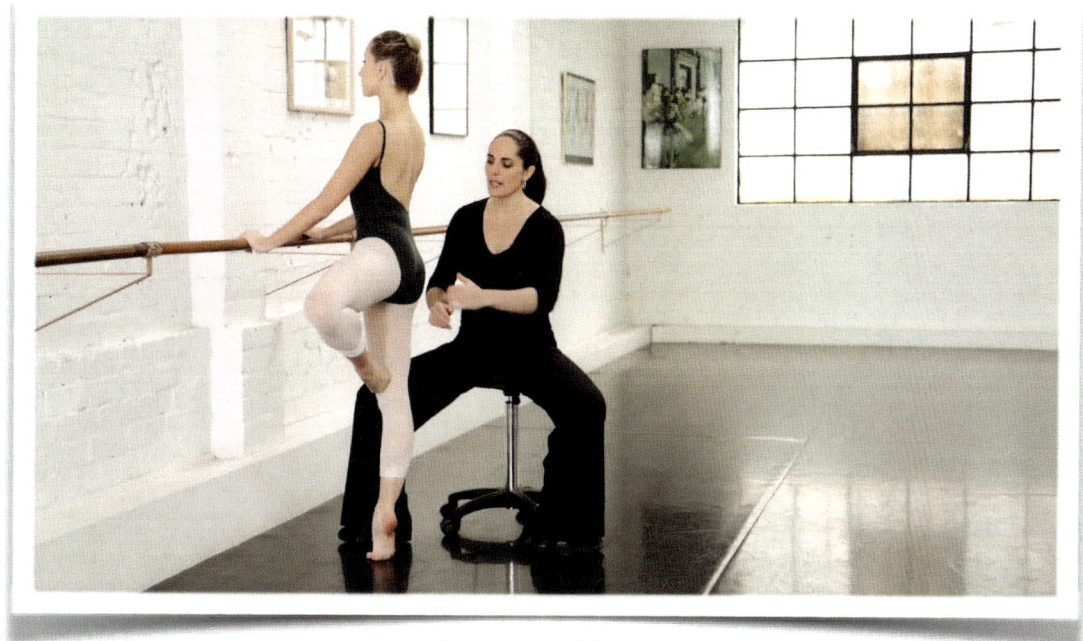

Pirouettes

One part of class that many dancers hate missing out on is pirouettes. However, as turning can place a lot of rotational and torsional strain on the foot it is one of the last parts of class that you will progress back to. Starting to turn too early can irritate an injury that is otherwise going well. However, while you are not turning this is a great time to work on:

- The rotational control of your core
- The alignment and control of your foot on demi point
- Endurance in your balance on demi point
- Control of the body on the supporting leg
- Proprioception in the injured foot

There are many exercises that could have been included in this section, so feel free to add any additional ones from our other programs that focus on these areas. Make sure to only progress from flat barre to work on rise and then on to turning with the approval of your therapist. When returning to class remember to include traditional pirouette exercises such as the 1/4, 1/2 and single turn exercise to improve your control in holding your pirouette position. Start with single turns in all your set exercises and focus on sustaining the balance at the end of the turn rather doing multiple turns.

Will I Ever DANCE Again?

Pirouettes - Foam Roller

One area that is really good to work on when you are not turning in class is the rotational stability of your core. Interestingly, a lot of dancers are not very good at this when I initially test them. A great way to do this is on a Foam Roller, as it is almost impossible to cheat! This exercise is great for training the deepest abdominal and back muscles as well as the obliques in a different way.

1. Start by lying lengthways on a long foam roller. Make sure that the spine is in neutral and the feet are together. Maintain a small lift under the low back but ensue that the front of the pelvis is horizontal and parallel to the floor.

2. Place your fingertips on your hip bones to check for any movement. In the early stages you can keep your elbows on the floor for balance, but as your stability improves you can try lifting them off the floor.

3. Lower one knee out to the side, making sure to keep both hips very still and facing the ceiling. Control the movement with the deep inner thighs. Slowly bring the leg back to the centre.

4. Repeat on the other side, making sure that the knee that is not moving stays pointing directly up towards the ceiling.

5. For a harder variation, take the arms into first position. Try lowering the opposite arm to the working leg out to the side. This exercises can be done with the injured foot in a boot, or with it taped.

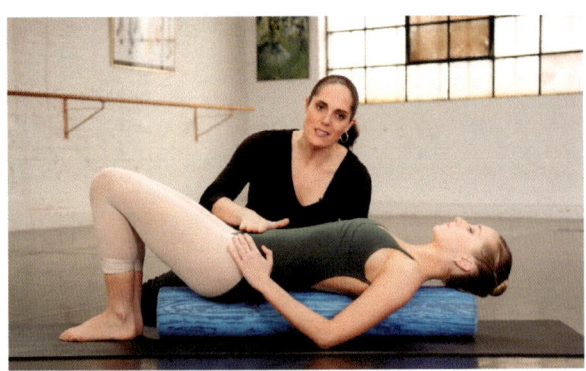

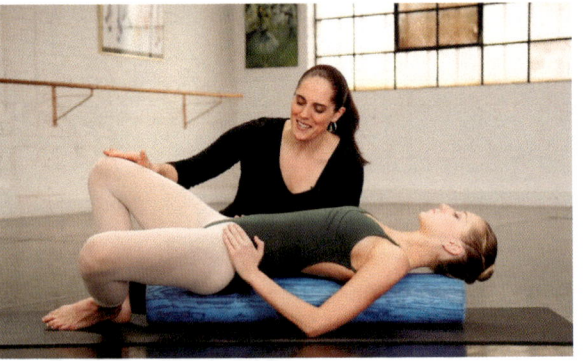

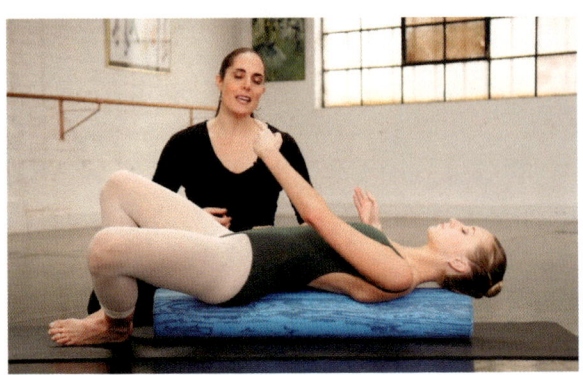

Will I Ever DANCE Again?

Pirouettes - Side to Side

Another way to challenge the rotational stability a little more is with this 'side to side' exercise. In this exercise we practice controlling the spine into rotation with several different positions of the legs to gradually increase the challenge. Please do not push yourself to do this too early. You must be able to comfortably maintain control of your deep abdominals with both feet off the floor to do this exercise.

1. Start by taking one foot, and then the other off the floor so that the shins come to be horizontal, parallel with the floor. Make sure to keep the deep abdominals on, slightly hollowing through the lowest part of the abdomen. If this is challenging for you, then please just practice this as an exercise before progressing.

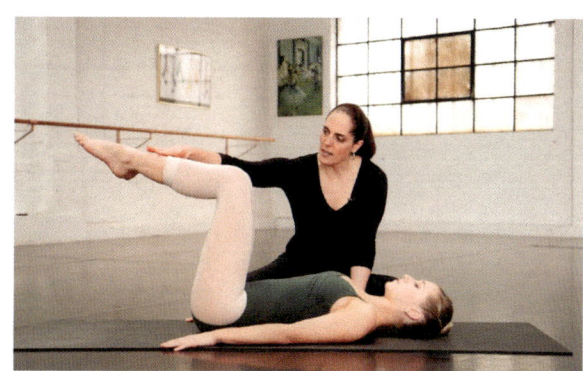

2. Keep the knees close together, and then lower both knees over to one side. Let the hip lift off the floor but keep the shoulders in contact with the floor and the chest relaxed.

3. Make sure that the spine is in neutral as you pass through the centre before repeating on the other side. Do not flatten the low back into the floor. This helps strengthen the deep stabilising muscles of the low back.

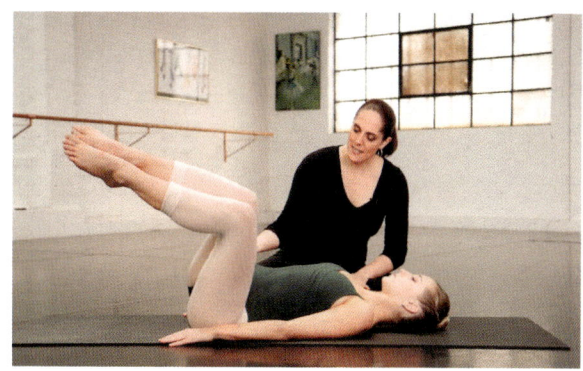

4. Repeat several times each side, keeping your breathing relaxed.

5. For greater challenge, lower the knees to one side, then straighten the legs before bringing the pelvis back into the centre. Make sure to maintain neutral spine. The added weight of the legs makes a big difference to the difficulty of the exercise.

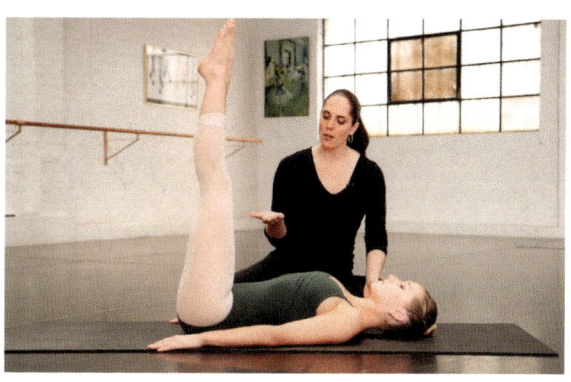

Will I Ever DANCE Again?

Pirouettes - Proprioceptive Exercises

For the final area while waiting to get back to turns, you should include some proprioceptive balance exercises. This is just a big word to describe your brain's ability to sense where your body is in space. If you have had a serious foot injury and been in a lot of pain, your brain can do an interesting thing where it drops its awareness of sensation in the foot in order not to feel so much pain. It is very important to retrain the brain's ability to feel the foot so that you can get your stability back for controlling your turns.

1. Start by standing in parallel with the feet very close together. Then try closing your eyes. This takes away the visual feedback that we often rely too much on.

2. Make sure to keep the weight slightly forward in the foot as if you were about to rise. It is ok to feel the tendons flicking on a little around the ankles as they attempt to stabilise the foot. You might be quite surprised at how difficult this is!

3. Next try taking one foot in front of the other, closing your eyes if you feel comfortable. Make sure to have something close by to hold onto if you lose your balance.

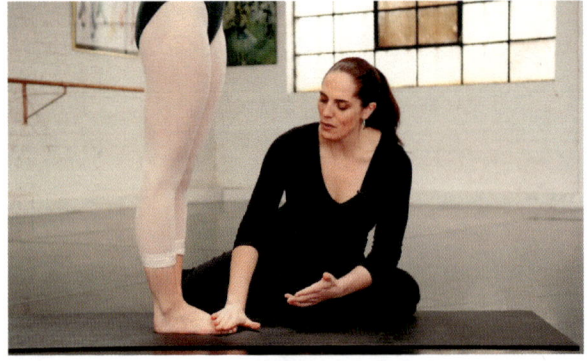

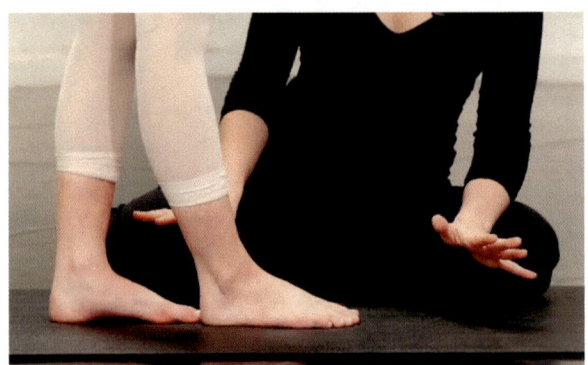

NB: This is a great exercise if you have ever noticed that you are much more unstable when performing a variation on stage, when the theatre is dark, compared to when you are in the studio. This is an indicator that you are using visual feedback, rather than an internal awareness of your body's placement to work out where you are in space. Practising your barre work with your eyes closed is another great way to increase your proprioception, and to really feel the music.

Will I Ever DANCE Again?

Pirouettes - Plié & Relevé for the Other Foot

While you are rehabilitating one foot it is important not to forget about the other foot! While you are not doing your normal turns and rises on the injured foot it is very important to continue strengthening the 'good' foot so that it does not lose condition. I do not like people with serious foot injuries doing turns on their non-injured foot due to the risk of falling out of the turn and landing awkwardly on the injured foot. Instead I usually recommend some exercises at the barre.

1. Standing at the barre, place the injured foot in a petit retiré position.

2. Slowly plié and rise on the non-injured side approximately 25 times. Try working with a rise initially, but you may progress this to a relevé as you gain more control.

3. Make sure to keep the hips level, facing the barre and keep the deep abdominals on. Control the turnout of the supporting leg so that the knee en fondu is aligned over the second toe of the supporting foot.

4. Once you are allowed to put weight through the injured foot you can try this exercise in first position (rising on two legs), and then slowly progressing to be able to do it on the injured side.

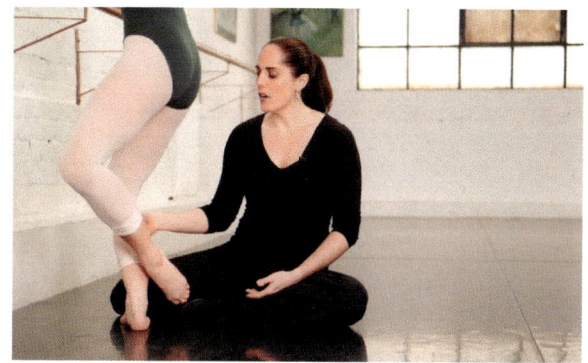

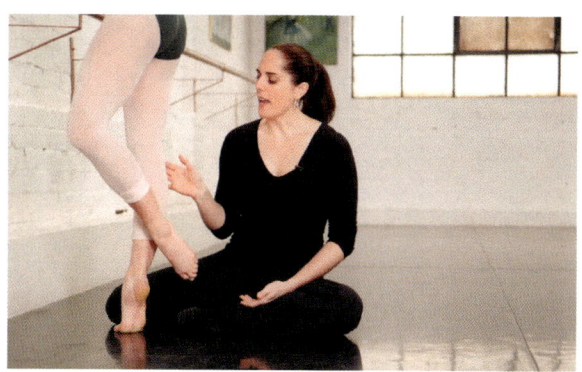

NB: There are many variations of this exercise that you can try, but make sure to only progress back to rising under the guidance of your therapist. There is no set timeframe even for people who have had the same operation or injury. Go at your own pace but challenge the non-injured leg. Some people worry that the 'good' leg will get "too far ahead" of the other one, but in fact the opposite is true. If the 'good' leg has been strengthened properly, it is faster for the brain to copy these instructions over to the injured side once there is no pain and you are allowed to put pressure on it again.

Will I Ever DANCE Again?

Pirouettes - Balance in Retiré

When you are starting to build the injured foot back into class for turns it is important to get your balance and placement right. You can start to do this even if you are not allowed to rise. For this exercise we will go through a simple preparation and then place the foot in a pirouette position keeping the supporting foot flat, and taking the hands off the barre to check your balance.

1. Start with the un-injured foot to the back in fifth position. Degagé to the back and then place the foot in a short fourth position as if you are preparing for a turn.

2. Bring the uninjured foot up to a pirouette position, but keep the supporting foot flat. Make sure the foot is in a tripod foot position, and the weight is slightly forward, rather than sinking through the heel.

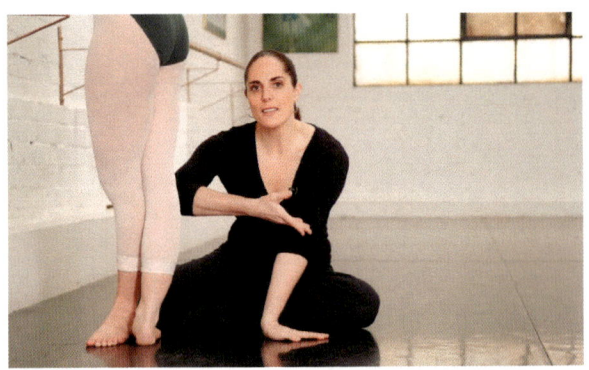

3. Take the hands off the barre, in a shortened first position as you would when you are turning. Balance for a few seconds, before placing the lifted foot back into a lunge, or as you would to finish a turn.

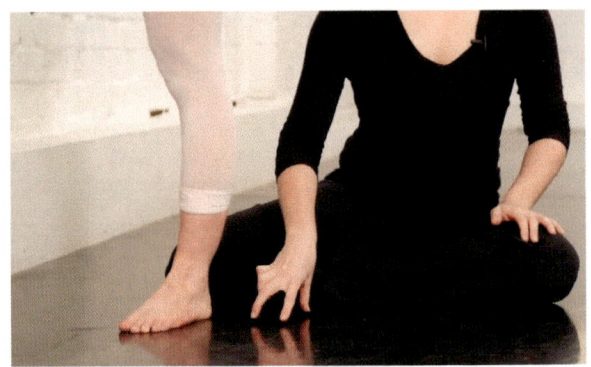

4. Once you are able to rise on the injured foot you need to start bringing this in to the balance. Focus on lifting through the arch and inside the ankle of the supporting foot.

5. Slowly increase the speed of the rise / relevé, and also increase the speed of taking the hands into first until you are able to do the relevé and hold in the centre.

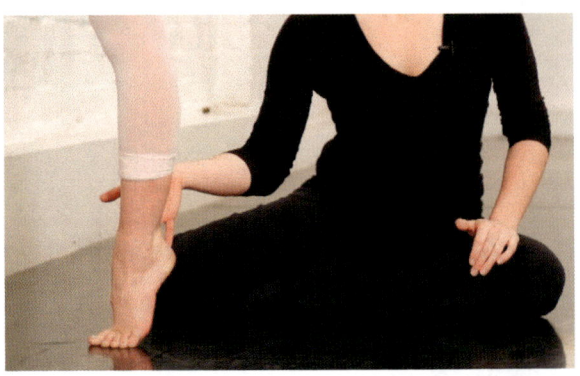

Will I Ever DANCE Again?

Pirouettes - Demi Point Balance

Once you can rise on the injured foot you need to start building back the endurance of the demi point position. Young dancers will only be able to cope with 10 seconds or so unsupported, but full time or pre-professional level dancers should be able to hold this balance for around 30 seconds before recommencing multiple turns.

1. Start in fifth with the un-injured foot in front.

2. Slowly rise in fifth, then draw the uninjured foot up into a pirouette position.

3. Once you have found your balance, try taking your hands off the barre and balance unsupported for as long as you can control your alignment. . Keep the knee pulled up and the toes long (not clawing)

4. Focus on keeping lifted through the arch of the supporting foot.

5. It is amazing how tired the calf will get in the early stages of practicing this exercise, however this is essential to build back this endurance before attempting multiple turns in the centre.

6. Make sure to build up your endurance in this exercises slowly, especially when recovering from any discomfort of surgery in the back of the ankle, (for example: Os trigonum removal, posterior impingement, pain in the Achilles or FHL tendinopathy) and always be guided by your therapists instructions.

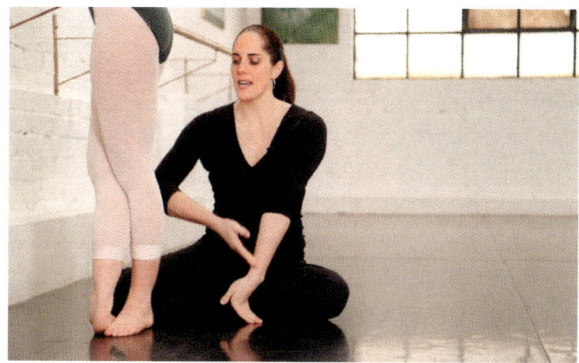

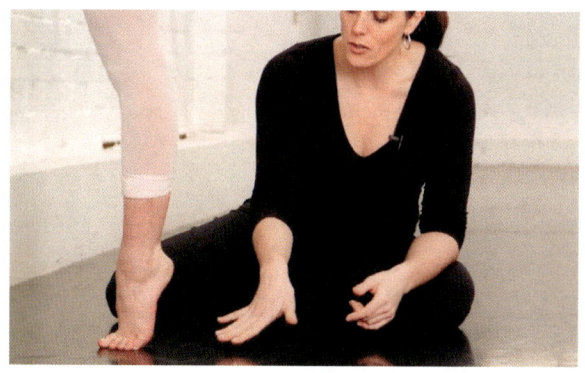

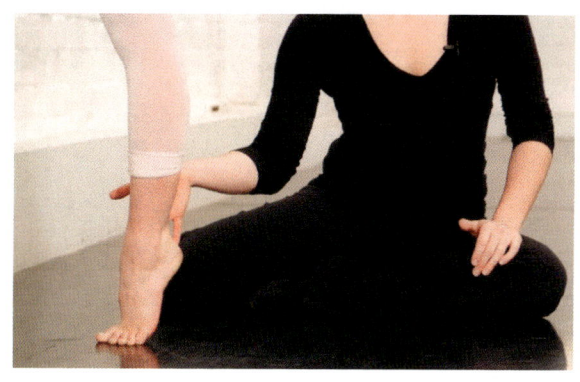

Will I Ever DANCE Again?

Pirouettes - Preparation for Pirouette

This exercise is a great way to challenge the hips, core and foot control at a higher level while waiting for the foot to fully heal and to prepare for recommencing advanced turns in the centre. It is a wonderful exercise to explore the subtleties of turnout control in different positions and helps avoid 'gripping' with the gluteals when controlling turnout. Remember to always be guided by your therapist as to how much of the exercise you can do on a rise.

1. Start with the feet in fifth position. Degagé the back leg and then plié in fourth, taking care to really keep both feet in a good position.

2. Do a slow rise on the front foot bringing the working leg into a pirouette position. Focus on careful placement of the supporting foot and on working the turnout at the top of the lifted leg.

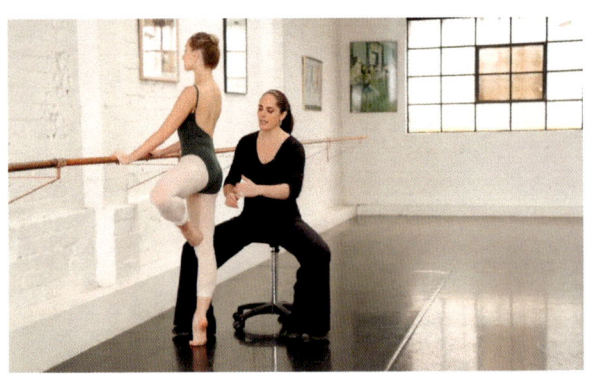

3. Unfold the working leg into attitude, then lower the supporting heel. Fondu, maintaining alignment of the knee over the supporting foot and keeping the lifted leg well placed in attitude.

4. Straighten both legs at the same time to come into an arabesque, and then rise on the supporting foot, maintaining the height of the lifted leg.

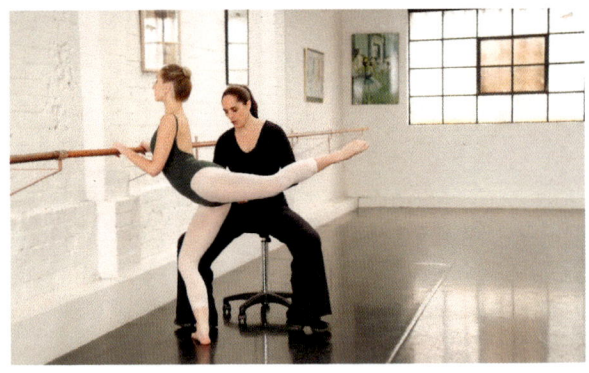

5. Maintaining the rise, bring the lifted leg into a pirouette position. Find your balance, then place the foot back into fourth, plié, then degagé and close.

6. Feel free to add in any balances with the hands off the barre if this is appropriate at your stage of rehab. This exercise can also be done on flat if you are not yet able to rise.

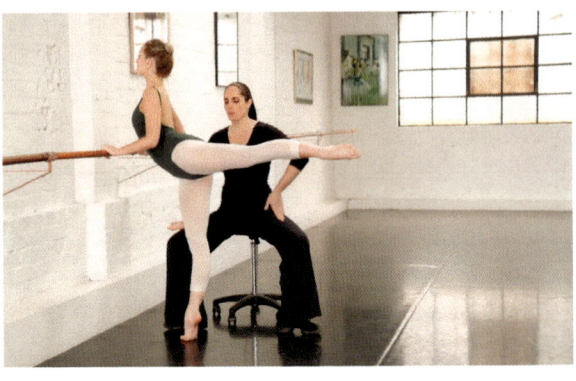

Will I Ever DANCE Again?

Allegro

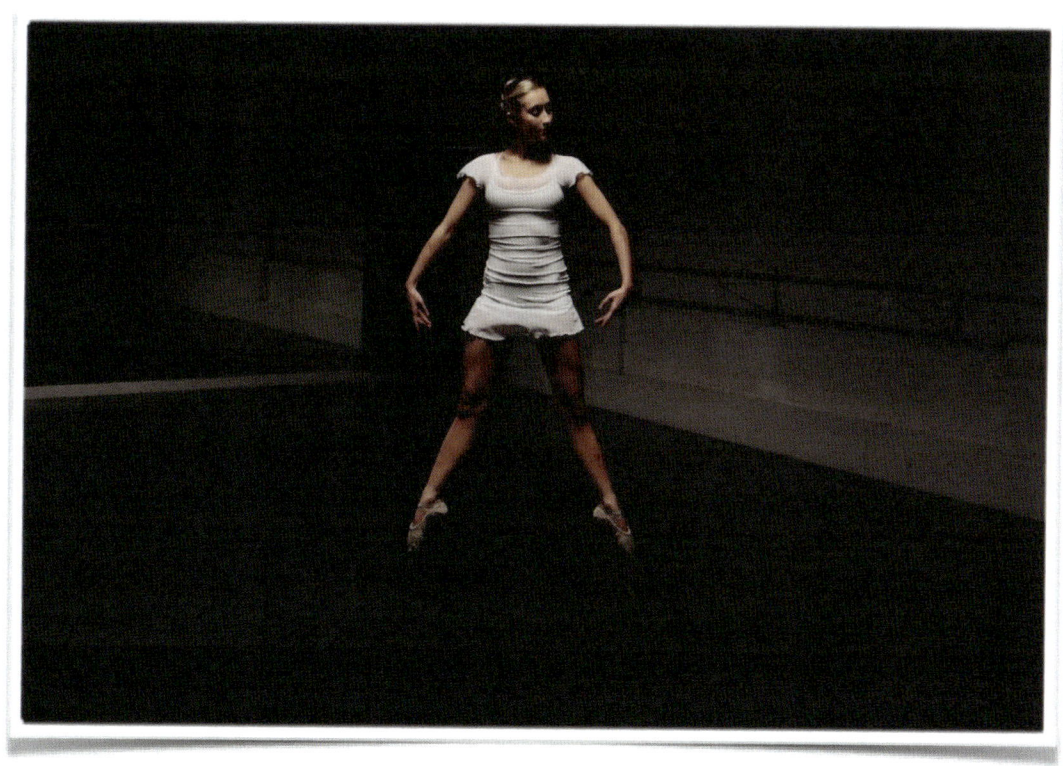

Will I Ever DANCE Again?

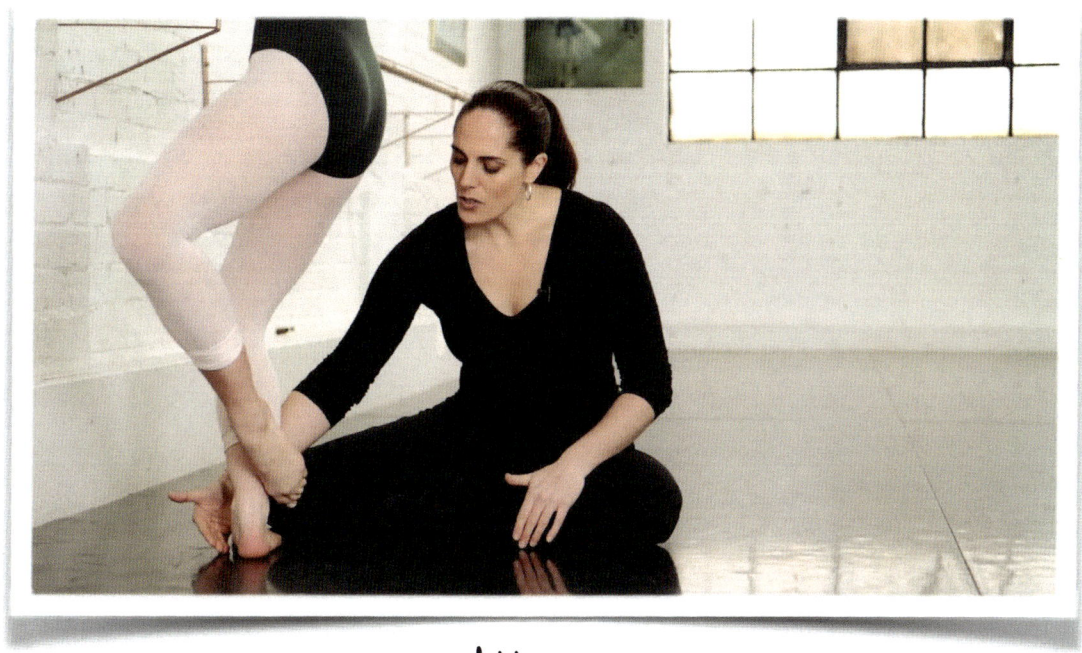

Allegro

A lot of people will be wondering about how you can work on your allegro or petit allegro when you are not allowed to walk, let alone jump on your foot. But there are actually lots of muscles that contribute to jumping properly that you can train before you actually get back into class.

One of these is actually the bottom part of your bottom, your Inferior Gluteal muscles. A lot of dancers focus on not using their bottom because they are trying to isolate their turnout muscles. It is true that your gluteals are not very effective turnout muscles and we should not use them for turning out, however you do need to use them for jumping.

There are many other components of allegro that you can work on while you are not allowed to jump on an injured foot or knee. These include: learning how to work through the feet on take off and landing, controlling the landing of a jump through the feet and controlling the alignment of the hip and leg with the turnout muscles, lateral stabilisers of the hip and deep core stabilisers.

It is extremely important to take any progressions in this section carefully and always be guided by your therapist as to which exercises are appropriate at certain points in your rehabilitation program.

Will I Ever DANCE Again?

Allegro - Gluteal Firing

It is important to make sure that the bottom part of the buttock is firing before you move into the other allegro exercises. One way to do this is to test how easily it comes on in a simple leg lift. If you can get this muscle working correctly it will take the load out of the hamstrings and lower back, and may even improve your flexibility!

1. If someone else is helping you test these muscles they will need to place their fingertips in your back muscles, the top of your bottom, the bottom of your bottom (right on the line of your leotard) and in your hamstrings.

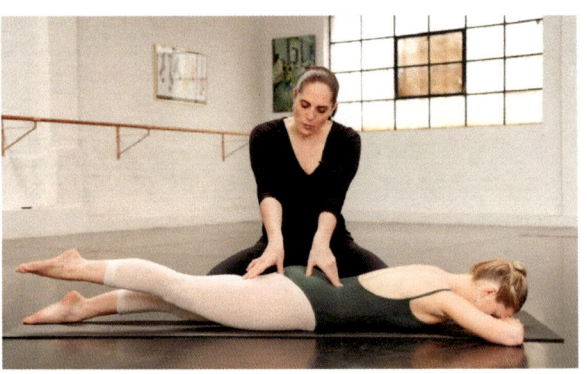

2. Once they have the position, lift your leg just off the floor. Your partner is wanting to feel if the inferior gluteal muscles work before the hamstrings do. Occasionally the gluteals will not work naturally and the bottom will stay relaxed. If this is the case it is something that you do need to retrain as the incorrect firing pattern can place a lot of load on both your low back muscles and your hamstrings.

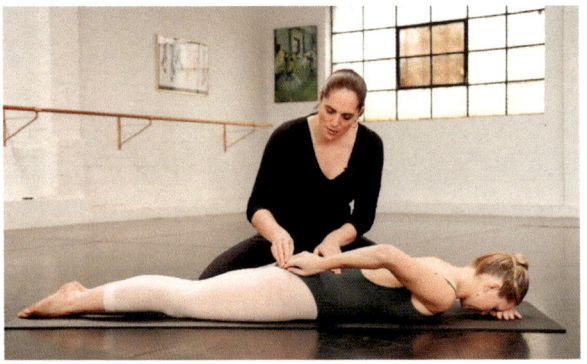

3. To retrain this, place your hand on the bottom part of your buttocks. Focus on gently contracting bottom part of the buttock. You should feel this muscle firm up underneath your fingers. Try to make it switch on before your hamstring muscles do.

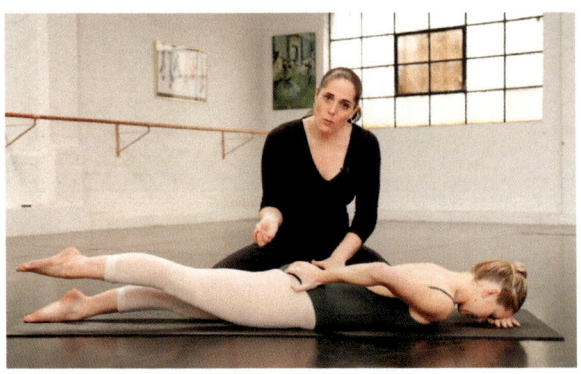

4. Slowly lift the leg using the inferior gluteals to take the weight out of the leg. Slowly lower the leg down and relax the gluteal muscle. Make sure to activate your core to reduce load into the back. Repeat 8 - 10 times until it starts to feel more natural.

Will I Ever DANCE Again?

Allegro - Heel Press into Ball

> Using a large ball for this exercise will create an unstable base which will challenge your hip stabilisers more. If you don't have a large ball you can use one of the small stability balls or the edge of a bed or sofa. Many dancers lose control of their low back when jumping, which wastes a lot of the kinetic energy that can help you jump. Improving the control of your gluteal muscles and your low back stabilisers at the same time is a wonderful way to keep your back and hips in condition for jumping.

1. Start with your spine in neutral, your core on and one foot up on the ball.

2. Slowly press your heel into the ball using the same inferior gluteal muscle as used in the previous exercise. Initially the ball will start to shake, but focus on stabilising the whole leg from the hip. As you get stronger the ball will shake less.

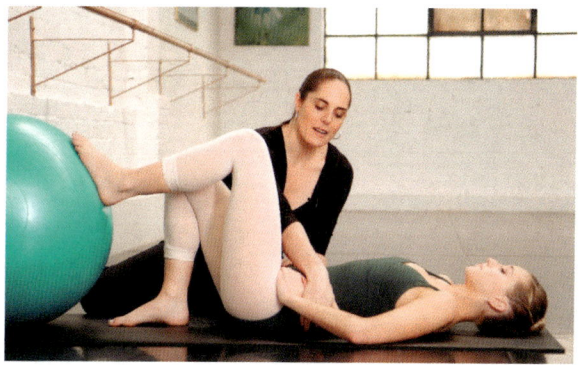

3. When you first start to do this you may feel that your lower back wants to flatten. This is due to weakness in the deep back muscles. Make sure to maintain the neutral spine position with the deepest back muscles, keeping the outer layers relaxed.

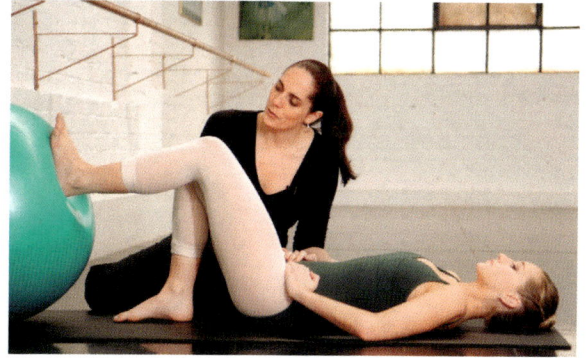

4. This exercise can also be done in your boot if you are not allowed to put weight through an unsupported foot.

5. Repeat the exercise in turnout, making sure that the knee is in line with the toe. This will help with your pliés as well as your jumps in turnout.

6. Do 10 - 15 repetitions of each variation, depending on your strength and endurance.

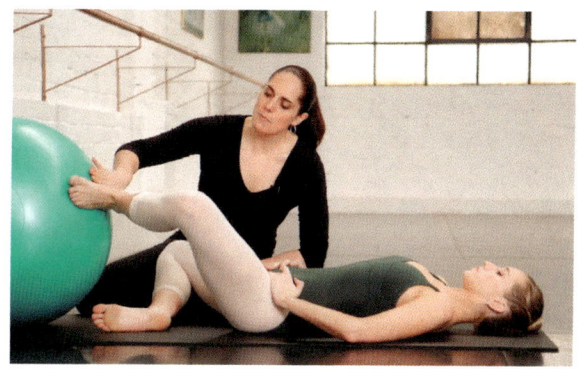

Will I Ever DANCE Again?

Allegro - Standing Jumps

Once you have found your deep gluteal muscles it is really important to learn how to use them when working back into your allegro. This exercise has three stages, and it is important in learning how to use the gluteals to cushion the landing of your jumps. This exercise helps take the load out of the front of the thighs and also helps re-pattern the appropriate sequence of muscles that should be used when jumping. Often this pattern is interrupted after having pain in the foot.

1. The first thing to master is the fondu. Stand onto one leg, feeling for the low gluteals along the line of the leotard. Slowly fondu, and use the gluteals to slowly allow you into the fondu (eccentric control). You should feel a gentle activation of the muscles as you fondu and also as you straighten the leg.

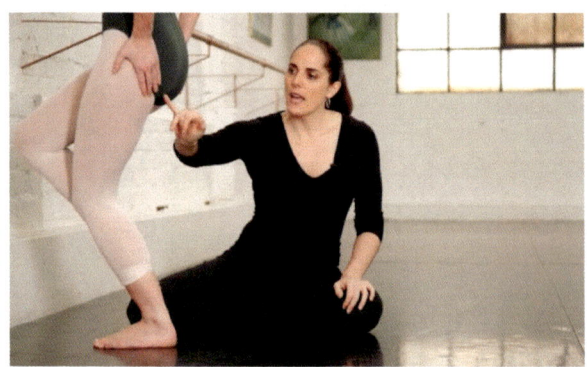

2. Make sure that you do not let the pelvis tuck as you fondu. This indicates weakness in the low back and gluteals.

3. For the second variation; fondu on the left, while working the right foot up through the demi point to be fully pointed off the floor as though you are jumping.

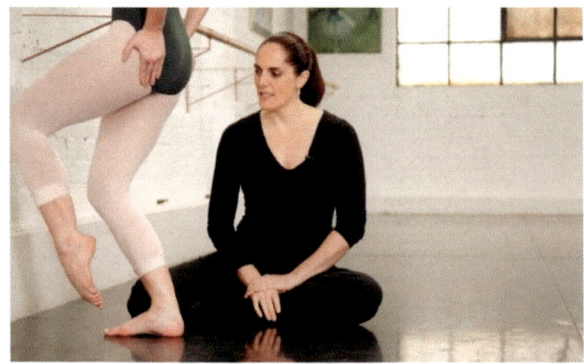

4. Make sure to keep the toes long, and to use the muscles that are used for the Doming and Toe Swapping exercises (as described in **The Perfect Pointe Book** and **Advanced Foot Control for Dancers** programs).

5. The third stage is to repeat this exercise in turnout. Start off in slightly less turnout than you would normally use to ensure good placement of the feet throughout.

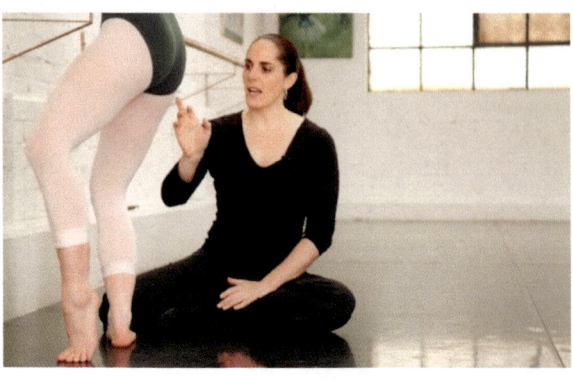

Will I Ever DANCE Again?

Allegro - Preparation For Petit Jeté

This exercise is a great way to prepare your feet for going back to the jumps in the centre. If you have done the **Advanced Foot Control** program you will know it's great training the Soleus muscle which helps cushion the landing of your jumps properly.

1. Start at the barre with your feet in first position. Use a little less turnout than you would normally use until you have the strength to control the position of your foot throughout the exercise.

2. Rise onto demi point, then transfer your weight onto one leg, slowly lowering the heel and moving en fondu at the same time.

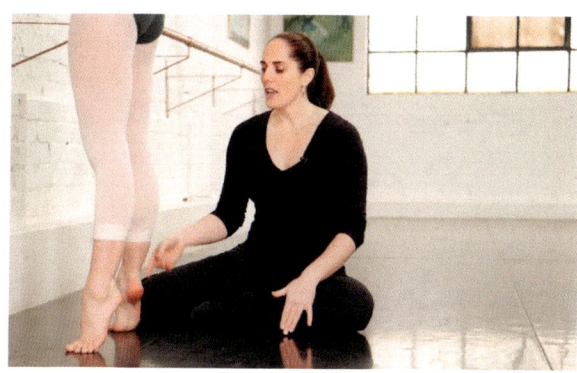

3. Rise back up on a single leg and repeat on the other side.

4. Remember to stay lifted through the arch of the foot as you lower into the fondu. Make sure you start bending the knee as you lower the heel, rather than lowering the heel and then bending the knee.

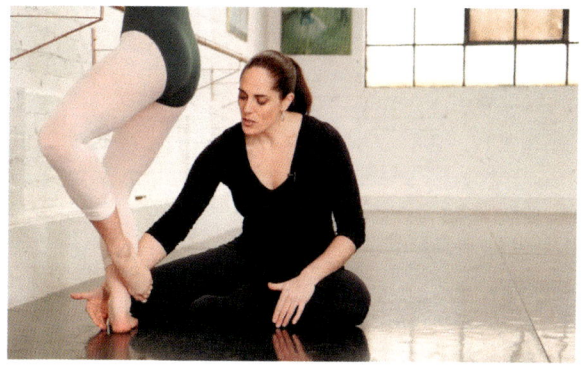

5. Remember to activate the deep turnout muscles consistently to keep correct alignment of the leg.

6. As your strength improves, and under the guidance of your therapist, you may start to increase the speed of this exercise. It is important to make sure that the 'memory' of this movement is almost automatic so that it is maintained when you start moving back to do jumps in the centre.

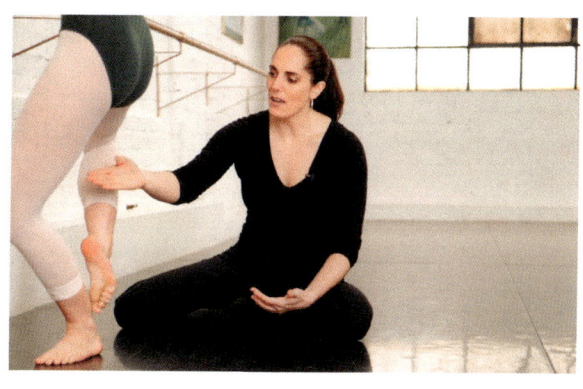

Will I Ever DANCE Again?

Allegro - Preparation for Grande Jeté

> The final exercise in this section is a preparation for a grande jeté. After a serious foot injury it does takes a while to build back to all of your grand allegro, but this is a way that you can actually work on all of the other components of this step without putting too much load through the foot. Make sure to adhere to any restrictions that your therapist has given you for this exercise. For instance, you may need to do it on flat with the foot flexed in the air for some foot injuries.

1. Start sideways on to the barre. Fondu on the supporting leg and lift the other leg to 90 degrees. Pause to check your placement. Make sure you stay lifted through the low back (neutral spine) but gently hollow the low abdominals at the same time. Make sure that the supporting leg remains turned out.

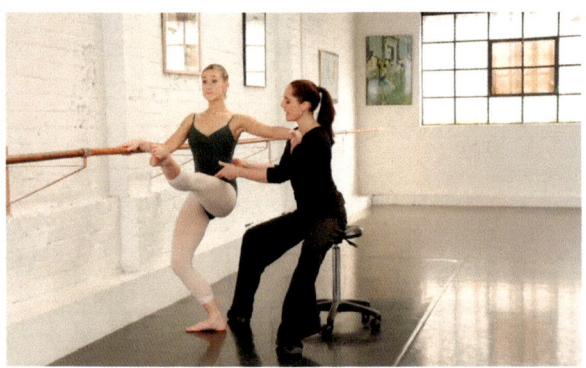

2. Rise on the back leg, travel through 4th position (on rise or flat) and then slowly lower into a fondu on the front leg, taking the back leg up to 90 degrees, keeping the chest lifted. Building the strength to maintain the leg horizontal to the floor is one of the biggest factors in achieving a beautiful line in the air.

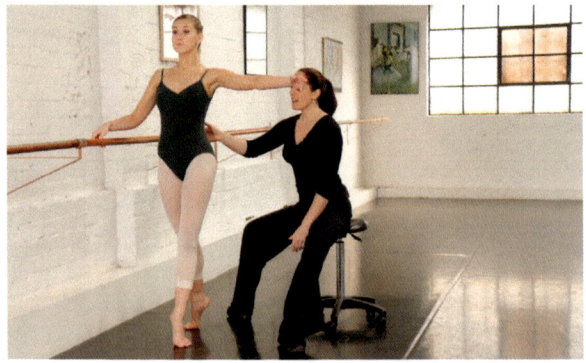

3. Transfer back through fourth position and then take the front leg up to 90 degrees again. Control the turnout on both the lifted and supporting legs from the deep turnout muscles in the back of the hips, taking care not to tuck the tail under.

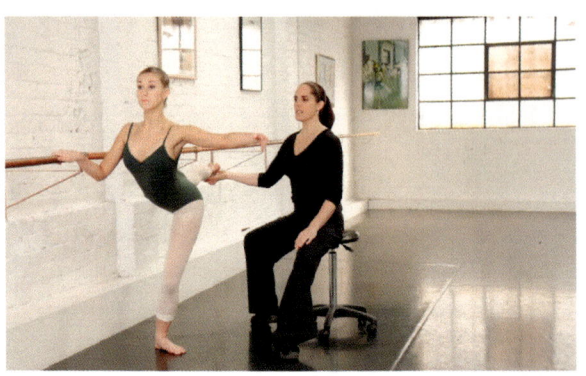

4. Repeat several times on each side. Once you have the pattern and positions established, speeding it up will make it more challenging before you progress to going back into the centre.

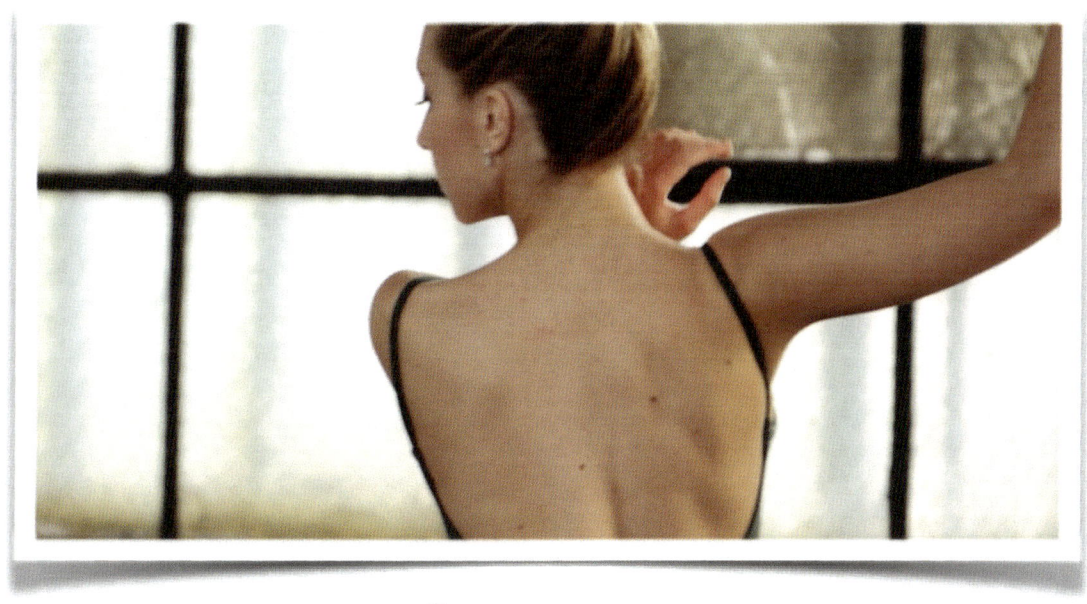

Getting Back Into Class...

Obviously – the progression back into class can be a personal one depending on the severity of the injury, and what contributing factors needed to be addressed. This is by no means a complete program for everyone who has a foot injury, and there are many other supporting exercises in all of our other programs to help keep you flexibility up, and your body working, while you allow the injury to heal.

Sometimes we need to let mother nature take her time – as was the case with Shay's injury. There are lots of things you can do to get healing happening as fast as possible - such as addressing your diet, and some forms of electro therapy, but it is important to give any ruptured or inflamed tissues time to heal. You may also be having hands on treatment which can radically improve the functionality of the foot, especially after being immobilised.

Returning fully to each section of class may take some time, depending on your injury. Please always follow your therapists advice whenever it comes to trying a new progression. Every injury, and every person is unique. Even dancers who had the same operation on the same day will progress at different rates so please do not try to compare yourself to anyone else as you move through your rehab.

Will I Ever DANCE Again?

1. **Non Weight-bearing** - This may include being taped, on crutches or in a boot, and in this stage you will want to restrict any pressure through the foot as much as possible.

   - Barre - Usually Floor Barre
   - Port de Bra - Seated
   - Adage - All floor work with the foot slightly floated off the floor
   - Allegro - Gluteal firing
   - Pirouettes - All floor work with feet off the floor
   - Pointe - None
   - Other Exercises - Make sure to do lots of core, turnout, spinal mobility exercises as well as intrinsic foot muscle exercises and single leg rises on your non injured foot.

2. **Weight-bearing on flat** - No Pointing or Rise - This is often when recovering from posterior ankle pain or surgery. Please do not rush this stage.

   - Barre - Usually Floor Barre or a flat barre with a flexed foot if an ideal foot position can be maintained (often just 2 - 3 exercises initially)
   - Port de Bra - Seated
   - Adage - All floor work, keeping foot flexed
   - Allegro - Gluteal Firing, Heel Press, Single Leg Fondu. Here you may be able to add in the first part of the Standing Jumps, but will not be able to point the feet. Syllabus work may be marked performing the plié part of each jump only.
   - Pirouettes - All floor work, Proprioceptive Exercises, Balance in Retiré, Preparation for Pirouette (on flat).
   - Pointe - Balance exercises in shoes on flat only.
   - Other Exercises - Continue with all exercises as above. You may also be able to do a lot of the self treatment massage techniques in the Advanced Foot Control for Dancers program.

Will I Ever DANCE Again?

3. **Weight-bearing - Pointed Foot** - Once you are allowed to point the foot, but not rise, you can add this in to the previous stage. For instance adding in the second stage of the Standing Jumps exercise. Also add in exercises such as Pointe Through the Demi Pointe from other programs.

4. **Weight-bearing - Double Leg Rise** - Once you are allowed to rise, this must be brought in slowly, with simple Plié / Rise combinations on two feet only.

   - Barre - Flat barre with double leg rises
   - Port de Bra - Standing
   - Adage - Syllabus exercises with legs low
   - Allegro - All floor work, Standing Jumps and a Plié / Rise combination on both feet.
   - Pirouettes - All previous work plus a double leg balance in first
   - Pointe - Seated Rises and flat barre work
   - Other Exercises - Make sure to do lots of Intrinsic Foot Muscle exercises, 3D Calf Stretches and self massage techniques on both feet

5. **Weight-bearing - Single Leg Rise** - Once you are allowed to rise, this must be brought in slowly, with simple Plié / Rise combinations on two feet only.

   - Barre - Normal Barre
   - Port de Bra - Normal Port de Bras
   - Adage - Syllabus exercises with legs at 90 degrees
   - Allegro - All previous exercises plus Preparation for Petit Jeté and Grande Jeté. Plié / Rise combinations on a single leg
   - Pirouettes - All previous work plus the Demi Pointe Balance and Preparation for Petit Jeté
   - Pointe - Double Leg Rises
   - Other Exercises - 3D Calf Stretches and self massage techniques as the calves can get tight when rebuilding endurance

Will I Ever DANCE Again?

6. Double Leg Jumps - Once you are allowed to jump, this must be brought in slowly, with simple two feet to two feet jumps only.

- Barre - Normal Barre
- Port de Bra - Normal Port de Bras
- Adage - Syllabus exercises with legs at full height (as foot control allows)
- Allegro - Jumps from two feet to two feet. I.e. Saute, Changement etc (no batterie or jumps taking off or landing on one foot). When the rest of the class is doing these exercises, work on the Preparation for Petit Jeté/Grand Jeté exercises.
- Pirouettes - Single Turns, plus the 1/4, 1/4, 1/2, 1/2, single turn combination.
- Pointe - Double Leg Rises with transfer to a single leg

7. Single Leg Jumps - Once you are allowed to start jumping and turning again it is wise to do just every second exercise in class in order not to fatigue the foot muscles too much. In between exercises you may do gentle stretches, mobilising exercises or gentle massage to keep the blood flowing.

8. Full Class - Do not be in a rush to get back to full class. Always take each day at a time, and gauge what to do in class based on how you feel, rather than what you 'should' be doing. Most people will have a flare up at some point when they accidentally do too much. DO NOT WORRY! Simply ice the foot, drop back 1 - 2 stages and begin to rebuild once the inflammation or pain has settled.

I do hope that you have enjoyed working through this program with us, and that it has given you lots of ideas about how to really make the most of your training time, and to return to class as strong as possible. From both Shay and I, thank you for sharing our story and we hope that your return to dance is as successful as hers has been!

Will I Ever DANCE Again?

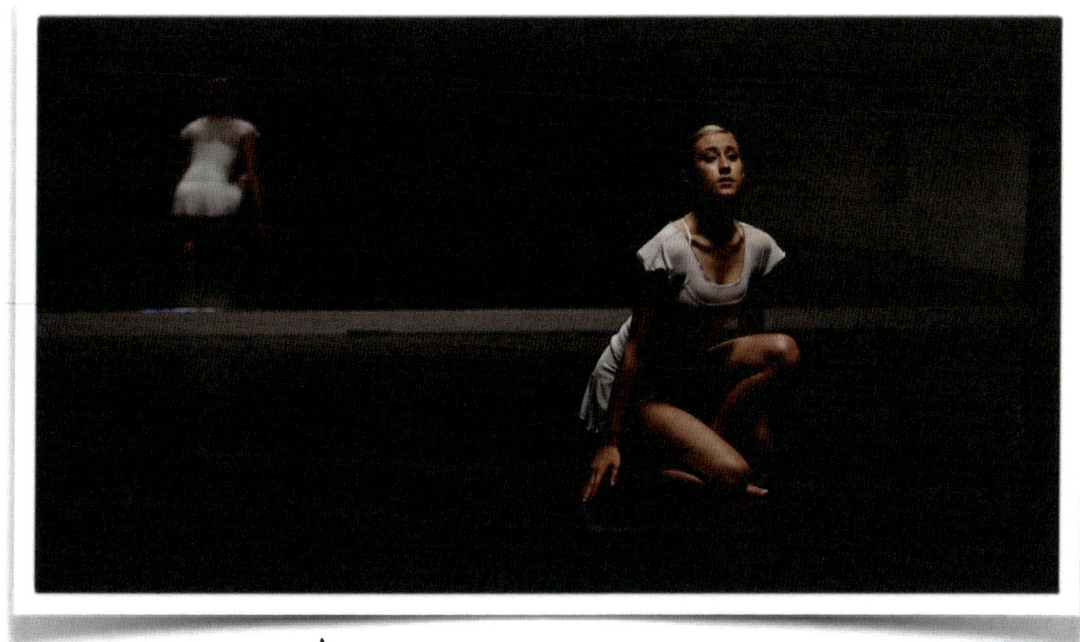

The Story Continues...

At the time we filmed the DVD of this program, Shay had been home for just three months. She had been in the boot (at gradually decreasing periods of time) for just over 2 months, and she had been out of it for just 3 weeks. To help her build back to performance level and watch her dance again was such a beautiful and fulfilling experience.

Shay then returned to full time training, and was even able to perform en pointe in a Gala event for Tanya Peason's 75th birthday several weeks after the DVD was filmed. This event was featured on "An Australian Story"

She is currently auditioning for a company position, and is dancing beautifully.

Her wish with the solo that she prepared for the filming of this DVD is to remind you never to give up. Even when diagnosed with an injury that could have ended her career, with the correct treatment, and very careful slow rehab, she was able to return to the path towards her dreams.

Will I Ever DANCE Again?

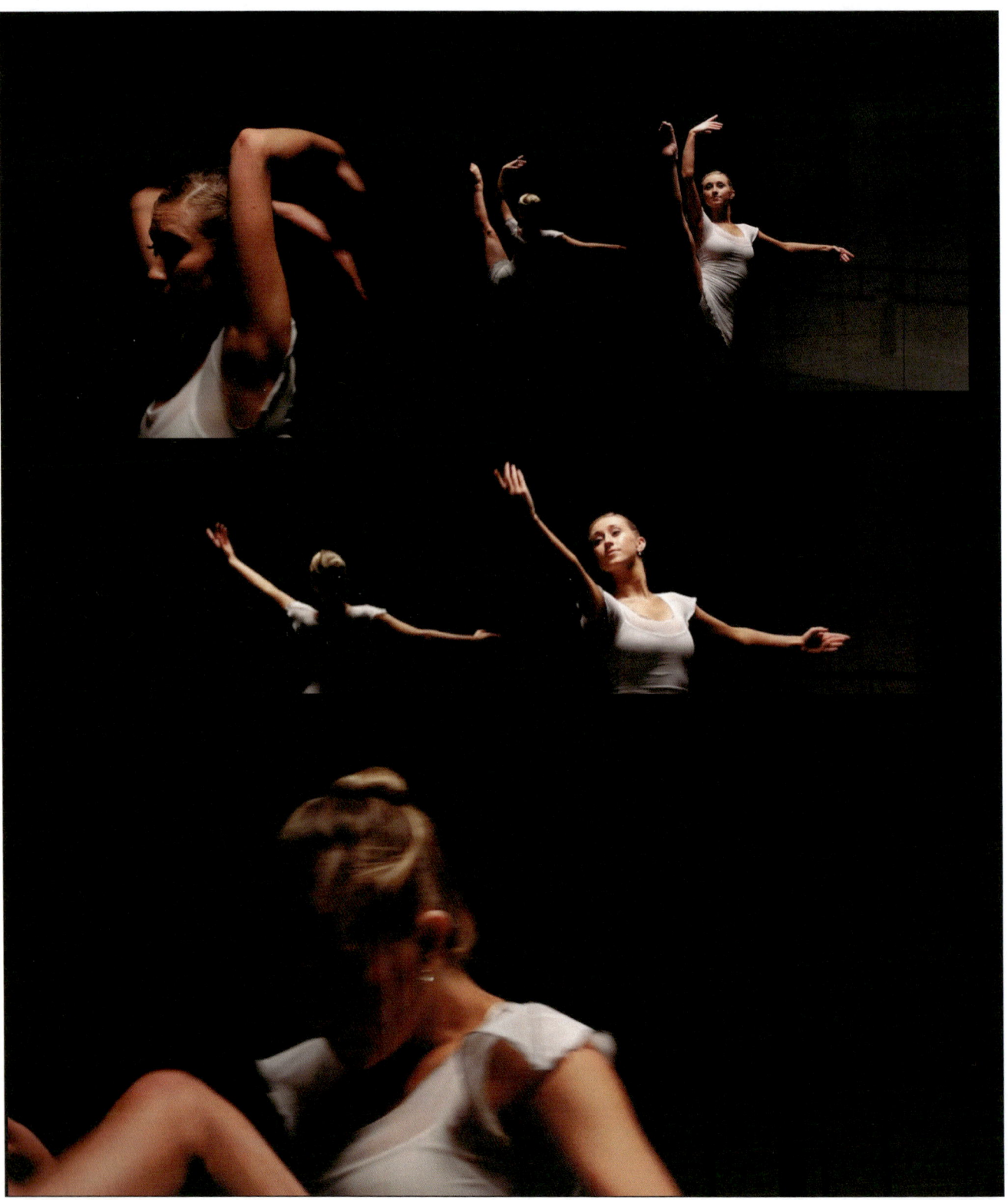

Will I Ever DANCE Again?

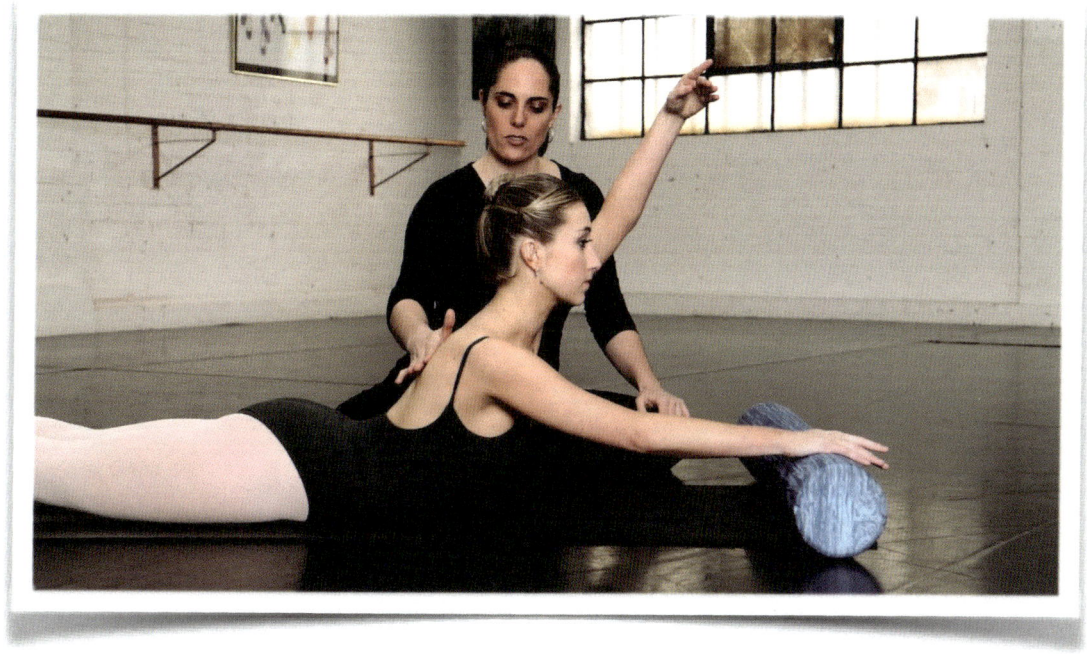

Equipment:

Foam Rollers: There are quite a few variations of Foam Rollers, some are more dense than others. I like a long firm foam roller about 25 cm in diameter, and you can this for a lot of different exercises in this section. A denser foam roller will stay in shape longer so look for a "closed cell" foam, rather than one with visible bubbles.

Small Stability Balls: The ball that we use for this is approximately 25cm in diameter. Inflate it to approximately 75 percent, rather than to full capacity.

Large Stability Ball: When inflating a large "swiss ball" that has been in a box inflate it to just 80 percent and then leave overnight to let the creases soften. Inflate to full capacity the following day.

Resistance Bands: There are a lot of different resistance bands on the market, all with different colours, densities and uses. I usually choose to use a light to medium density band cut to 1.8 metres so that there is a lot to work with. You can then double the band over if you need more resistance.

Will I Ever DANCE Again?

Other Resources:

The Perfect Pointe Book

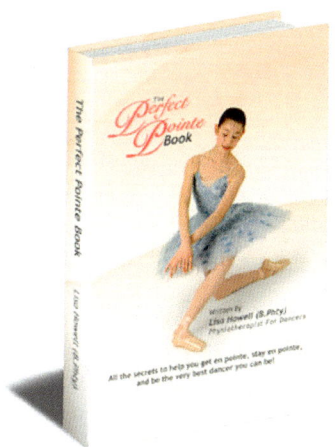

"The Perfect Pointe Book' rapidly became the bible for many students preparing to get en pointe after its release in 2005. Join the thousands of dancers and dance teachers all over the world who are relishing the opportunity to use this newly revised resource to ensure that all students are correctly prepared for pointe work.

The 118 page manual, and video tutorials are full of fabulous photographs and detailed instructions to ensure correct performance of all exercises. Written in clear simple terms, the program is divided into four easy-to-follow stages to work on:

- Mobility of the feet and ankles
- Strength of the inner foot muscles
- Turnout control
- Core control

Visit **www.theperfectpointebook.com** to download a free report on "The Top 10 Questions about starting en pointe"

The Perfect Pointe System
Pre-Pointe Assessment and Teachers Training Manual

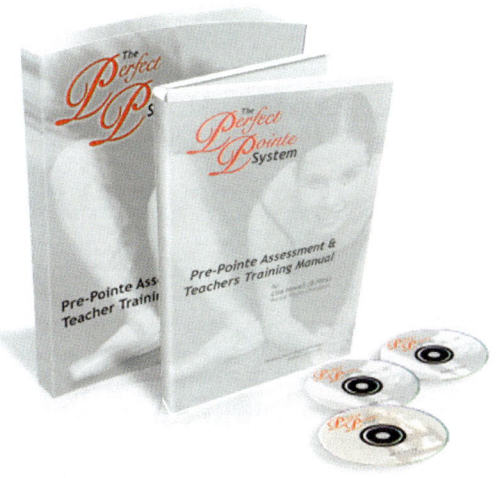

Are you concerned at just how well prepared your young students are when they progress onto pointe? Do you have students with repetitive strain or chronic injuries in the feet and ankles?

'The Perfect Pointe System' takes the science of dance medicine off the text book and into the classroom! Enjoy the combination of anatomical and scientific research in a clear and easy to use format to transform your teaching of pointe work to young students.

Learn the process of a detailed pre-pointe assessment, and also develop the understanding of how to read each test in a way that illuminates your understanding of the dancers' body.

The Perfect Pointe System encompasses a fabulous 130 page reference manual that provides formal assessment sheets and explains each test in detail, and also includes:

- Wall charts for easy reference
- Details of class plans to provide integration of the course into class work.
- Access to over 30 audio recordings discussing the finer points of each assessment test to further enhance understanding.

Visit **www.theteachersmanual.com** to learn more!

Will I Ever DANCE Again?

My Beginner Pointe

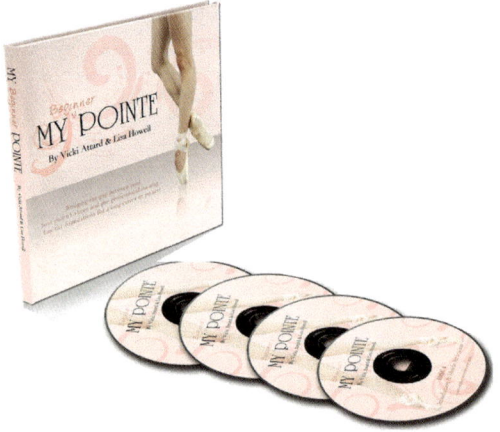

For the My Beginner Pointe program Lisa Howell teamed up with Principal Artiste, Vicki Attard to present a unique program which covers safe dance practices and aesthetic components, that combine to create successful classical dancers.

This comprehensive program includes three DVD's covering preparatory and strengthening exercises for pointe work, as well as three carefully choreographed stages of class work, providing a wealth of information in an uncomplicated format.

The program takes a young dancer from choosing their first pair of pointe shoes, through preparatory exercises and beginner class exercises, all the way to turns en pointe. The Audio CD completes the set; making the class work easy to practice at home or in the studio.

For more information, and to download your free video about "My First Pointe Shoes" visit http://mybeginnerpointe.com

The Perfect Pointe Parents Manual

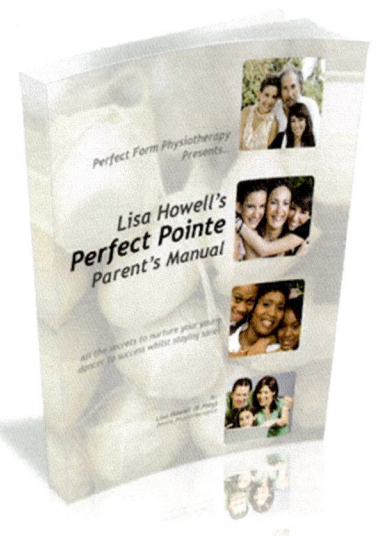

Do your dancers' parents assist your teaching or do they get in the way? Do they constantly ask you questions that you do not have the time to answer properly over and over again? Many parents are bewildered by the whole experience that is the dance world, and are often at a loss at how best to support their children. Whether this is in regard to nutrition, training techniques or emotional coping strategies in times of stress.

This manual answers all of these questions and more, and best of all - **it's FREE!**

Despite the insistence of everyone who has managed to get a sneak preview of it that I should be charging for it, I wanted to keep it free. I wanted to make sure that there was no barrier to any parent wherever they are in the world, no matter what the conversion rate is, to be able to access quality information that they can trust, in regards to learning the best things for their children.

"A thoroughly intelligent and well written work, answering all of the questions that parents seek answers to, as well as what they should know but don't think to ask!"

To download, visit http://www.theballetblog.com/shop/the-perfect-pointe-parents-manual-downloadable-ebook/

Will I Ever DANCE Again?

Advanced Foot Control for Dancers

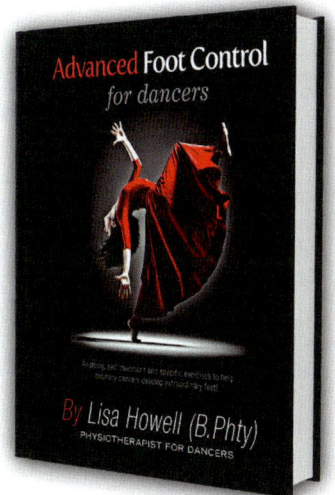

The Advanced Foot Control Program explores the anatomy of a dancer's foot – in the way a dancer needs to know it! The new revised edition features a full colour book and over 3 hours of accompanying online video.

1. A hard copy of the new Advanced Foot Control Book!

This 90 page full colour book has been completely revised, with full colour illustrations throughout to demonstrate all of the exercises and treatment techniques in the program clearly. The book will be delivered to your door and is a great resource for any serious dance student.

2. Instant access to 10 MP4 Videos

Over 2 hours of total playing time with each video exploring one of the major muscles in the lower leg in detail. Looking at the anatomy from a dancer's point of view and explaining all of exercises, massage techniques and stretches in MP4 format so you can either watch them online, or download them to your iPod.

3. Special Injury Reports

We have also created many Injury Reports and Bonus Taping Videos and PDFs, that help you understand common injuries. These essential reports outline everything you need to know about all of the most common dance injuries, including information on why the injury usually occurs, treatment options, what to avoid and how to progress back into class; as well as information for your therapist about the demands of a full recovery.

www.advancedfootcontrol.com

Injury Reports

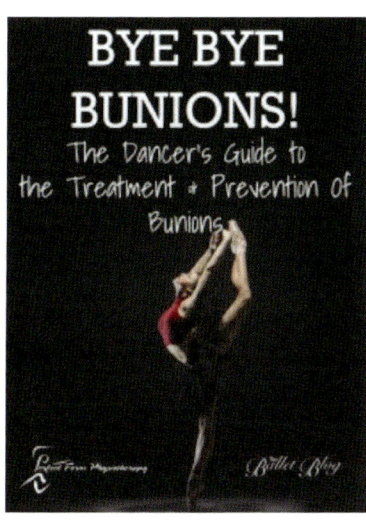

The foot and ankle injury reports that come with the Advanced Foot Control for Dancers program can also be purchased separately, along with injury reports on common issues with the hip, back and knee. These injury reports includes lots of information on common causes of injuries that often plague dancers. They include corrective exercises and treatment techniques to settle your pain as soon as possible. They also include information on how to structure a graded progression back into class and tips to help prevent the injury from coming back.

All of the foot and ankle injury reports are included in the Advanced Foot Control Member's Area on The Ballet Blog. If you are a member, please login and click on the member's area tab to view.

To view the selection of injury reports that we have created, visit
http://www.theballetblog.com/product-category/injury-rehab/

Will I Ever DANCE Again?

Front Splits Fast

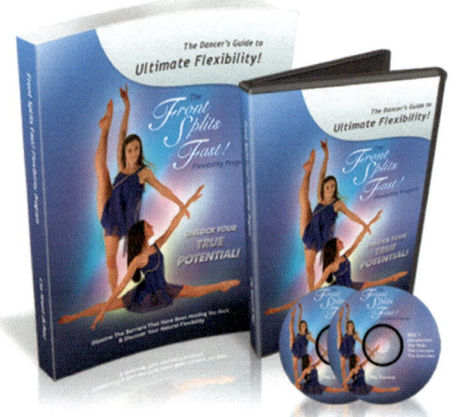

Getting into the splits comfortably is a dream for many dancers, as we never want our artistry to be limited by our mobility! This cutting edge program will help you to reach your dreams! This new edition includes a professionally recorded double DVD set with even more secrets to increase your flexibility! Many people struggle with regular stretching as it does not specifically address the true causes of their restricted mobility! Front Splits Fast is a revolutionary program which focuses on releasing one's neural and fascial tension to dramatically increase mobility throughout their body.

"I purchased this book about six months ago now and I love it! I am a late starter to dance so I needed to find a quick way to gain flexibility in the shortest amount of time. Within a month I was flat on both legs after doing the program every second day. I was amazed at how easy it really is! Now I do the program 1-2 times a week and incorporate my own stretches on a daily basis. Thanks Lisa for designing such an amazing program!" (Maddison)

For more information and to download our free "5 Myths about Flexibility" PDF please visit

[www.frontsplitsfast.com.](www.frontsplitsfast.com)

Core Stability for Dancers

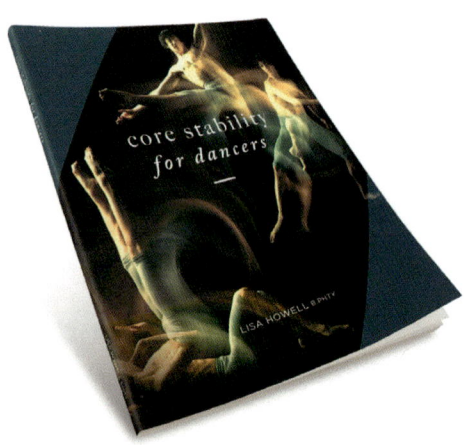

Most core training addresses the big 'global movement' muscles. While these muscles are important for any dancer, true core strength is more subtle and comes from much deeper within. This course addresses how to use true core control; how to train the right muscles and how to apply this to your dancing.

The aim of this Core Stability course is to achieve dynamic and fluid control of the spine, helping to attain higher extensions, better turns and relieve back pain. The course includes exercises to work on finding your neutral spine, strengthen your inner and outer unit muscles, as well as teach you how to activate you core while dancing! This book is essential training for any dancer or dance teacher wanting to take their dancing to the next level.

The process is split into several stages to allow each dancer to work at their own level, and gradually develop core stability in all directions, and with movement.

For more information please visit:

http://www.theballetblog.com/shop/core-stability-course-for-dancers

Will I Ever DANCE Again?

Training Turnout

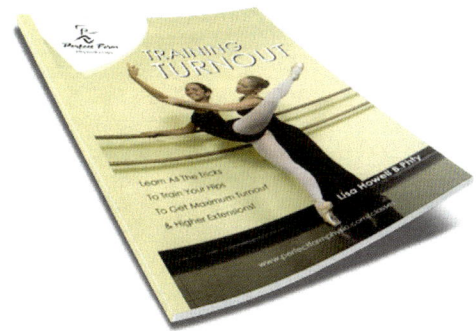

Our unique Training Turnout program covers the anatomy of the dancers' hip in an easy to understand way. It shows many different release techniques to improve range of motion, as well s how to work out exactly where you are restricted.

There are also progressive exercises to train all of the important muscles involved in great hip control. An essential resource for any dancer!

"I brought this book about six months ago because I was told that I had very tight hips and didn't know how to control my turnout. I was at a lost trying so many different products but nothing ever really worked. Often I would stretch out my hips so much to the point were I couldn't walk the next day. As soon as a brought the book I started to realise how much damage I am doing to my hips. The book helped me locate where my tension was and how to release it. Now before every class I bring my tennis ball with me to go through a couple of exercises and then everyday do some of the strength exercises. All of my teachers have told me what an improvement I have made. Thanks Lisa!" (Madison)

For more information please visit:

http://www.theballetblog.com/shop/training-turnout-manual/

Ball Conditioning for Dancers

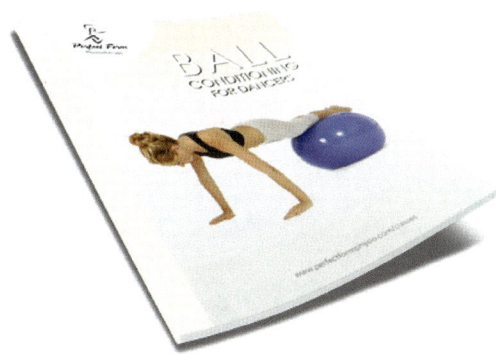

A large exercise ball can be a dancers' best friend and is wonderful for assisting in developing deep core strength, however many people do not know how to use a ball properly.

This course starts with the basics of core control and progresses to advanced exercises in an easy to follow way. There are two distinct levels of training, which is ideal for teachers bringing the exercises into a large studio.

With over 70 different exercises to challenge every student, this book helps teachers come up with interesting new ways to include in conditioning classes.

Students love working with equipment, and many of them will have a large stability ball at home, often lying around unused. This program will help to get them inspired to continue their core work independently.

For more information please visit:

http://www.theballetblog.com/shop/ball-conditioning-for-dancers/

Will I Ever DANCE Again?

Dance Conditioning One

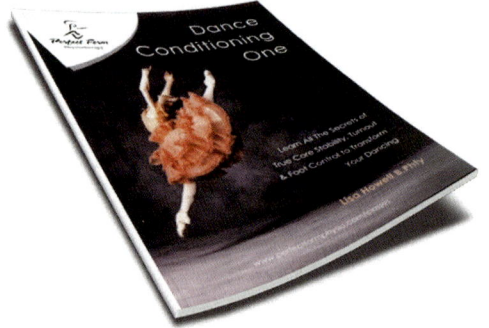

Our Dance Conditioning - Level One program is a wonderful collection of exercises and releases for beginner and intermediate dance students. Ideally suited for those dancers under the age of 16 years or adult students with less than four years training. This program includes a range of Pilates and Yoga based exercises specifically geared towards improving your core stability, turnout and some foot work specifically for dance.

This is an ideal resource for male students and those not interested in pointe work to develop a sensitivity and control of all areas of the body.

For more information please visit:

http://www.theballetblog.com/shop/dance-conditioning-one/

Dance Conditioning Two

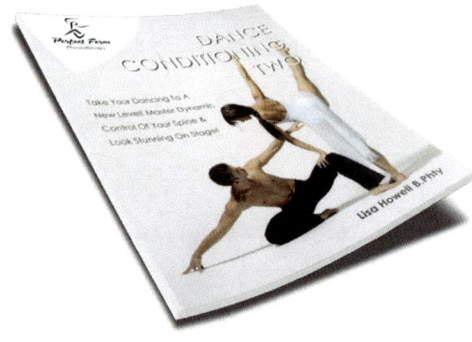

Our Dance Conditioning - Level Two program is a detailed collection of more advanced exercises to take your training to the next level. This program expands on the underlying knowledge gained in 'The Perfect Pointe Book' and 'Core Stability Course For Dancers' to provide a comprehensive training program suited for high level dancers.

This program was developed to give our higher level dancers a summary of all of the other programs to take away with them when they went overseas. It also helps them learn how to create their own ongoing rehab program, to keep it interesting.

For more information please visit:

http://www.theballetblog.com/shop/dance-conditioning-two/

Will I Ever DANCE Again?

www.PerfectFormPhysio.com.au

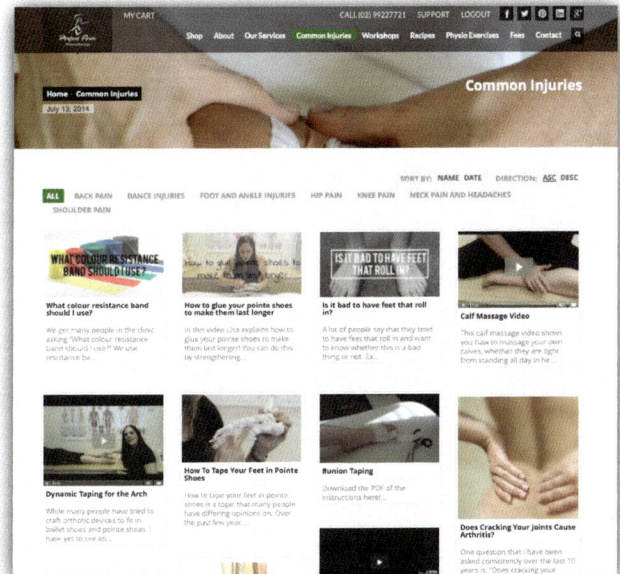

Perfect Form Physio was started by Lisa Howell in 2005 with the aim of giving dancers the highest possible level of care, in a nurturing environment. We are a specialised Dance Physiotherapy clinic and have worked with many different body types and styles of dance.

Knowing exactly what is physically demanded of you in each of these styles is so important in order to treat both dance students and professionals effectively. All of our therapists have a strong background and love for dance with good grounding in a variety of different dance styles.

Our aim is to change the world of dance by providing educational workshops and products for dancers, teachers and health professionals to prevent and reduce injuries by increasing the quality of the services given to dancers all over the world.

www.perfectformphysio.com.au

www.TheBalletBlog.com

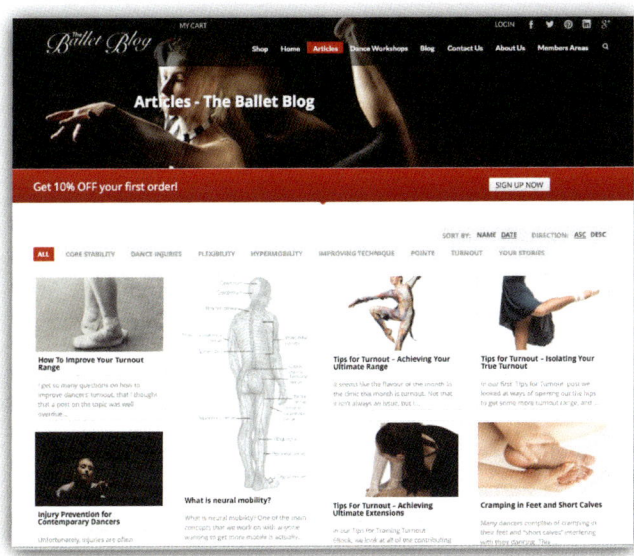

There is no better way to accelerate your dancing than mastering your own body! After success in developing **Perfect Form Physiotherapy,** a clinic for dancers of all disciplines in Sydney, Australia, we wanted an online portal to be able to help dancers worldwide. So, in 2007, The Ballet Blog was born!

The Ballet Blog website is dedicated to all dancers, dance teachers and students, giving you all of the tools and information you need to prevent and recover from injury as well as accelerate your technique to become the best dancer you can be! We have written hundreds of articles and filmed many videos to help you do this.

Sign up to our free weekly newsletter to get all the latest delivered right to your inbox.

www.theballetblog.com

Made in the USA
Charleston, SC
30 July 2014